A CLOSER LOOK AT WOUND INFECTIONS AND HEALING

NEW DEVELOPMENTS IN MEDICAL RESEARCH

Additional books and e-books in this series can be found
on Nova's website under the Series tab.

NEW DEVELOPMENTS IN MEDICAL RESEARCH

A CLOSER LOOK AT WOUND INFECTIONS AND HEALING

JOSEPH E. KEEL
EDITOR

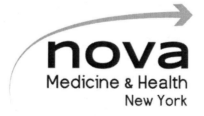

nova
Medicine & Health
New York

We have partnered with Copyright Clearance Center to make it easy for you to obtain permissions to reuse content from this publication. Simply navigate to this publication's page on Nova's website and locate the "Get Permission" button below the title description. This button is linked directly to the title's permission page on copyright.com. Alternatively, you can visit copyright.com and search by title, ISBN, or ISSN.

For further questions about using the service on copyright.com, please contact:
Copyright Clearance Center
Phone: +1-(978) 750-8400   Fax: +1-(978) 750-4470   E-mail: info@copyright.com.

NOTICE TO THE READER

The Publisher has taken reasonable care in the preparation of this book, but makes no expressed or implied warranty of any kind and assumes no responsibility for any errors or omissions. No liability is assumed for incidental or consequential damages in connection with or arising out of information contained in this book. The Publisher shall not be liable for any special, consequential, or exemplary damages resulting, in whole or in part, from the readers' use of, or reliance upon, this material. Any parts of this book based on government reports are so indicated and copyright is claimed for those parts to the extent applicable to compilations of such works.

Independent verification should be sought for any data, advice or recommendations contained in this book. In addition, no responsibility is assumed by the Publisher for any injury and/or damage to persons or property arising from any methods, products, instructions, ideas or otherwise contained in this publication.

This publication is designed to provide accurate and authoritative information with regard to the subject matter covered herein. It is sold with the clear understanding that the Publisher is not engaged in rendering legal or any other professional services. If legal or any other expert assistance is required, the services of a competent person should be sought. FROM A DECLARATION OF PARTICIPANTS JOINTLY ADOPTED BY A COMMITTEE OF THE AMERICAN BAR ASSOCIATION AND A COMMITTEE OF PUBLISHERS.

Additional color graphics may be available in the e-book version of this book.

Library of Congress Cataloging-in-Publication Data

ISBN: 978-1-53616-816-7

Published by Nova Science Publishers, Inc. † New York

CONTENTS

PREFACE

Wound healing is a complex cascade of events that led to reconstruct a damaged tissue with cellular and biological mechanisms. A Closer Look at Wound Infections and Healing first reviews the treatments mentioned in traditional Iranian medicine sources for various wounds.

The various antibiotic alternative therapies that could be used against antimicrobial resistant bacteria in wound infections are reviewed in detail.

The authors report on the complex role of estrogens and estrogenic derivatives in the wound healing process, with a focus on their therapeutic uses.

The penultimate chapter explores the impact of photobiomodulation therapy on wound healing and the basic biochemical reactions involved. Photobiomodulation therapy involves the use of low-powered light emitting diodes, lasers or broadband light, mostly in the visible red and near infrared light spectrum.

Postoperative surgical wound infection in the lumbar spine is unfortunately a common and potentially devastating complication. It is associated with increased morbidity and the need for further surgery. The authors discuss treatment of surgical wound infection centered on surgical debridement.

Chapter 1 - Wound healing is a complex cascade of events that led to reconstruct a damaged tissue with cellular and biological mechanisms.

Along with chemical drugs, in some case, herbal remedies work better and with fewer side effects. Almost 30% of traditional drugs applied to dermal disturbance and wound, while, only 1-3% of modern drugs are allocated to this goal. Traditional Iranian Medicine (TIM) is a rich knowledge source based on herbal drugs for treating diseases including treatment of various wounds. In TIM, wound in general has been known as Tafarrogh-e-ettesal that means tissue disconnection, which includes different wounds: Scratch (*kharash*): a superficial wound that cause damage only to the skin. Wound or injury (*jerahat*): a wound that in addition to the skin caused damage to its underlying tissue, but it is not infectious. In TIM, this type of wound divided into 10 subgroups. Sore or ulcer (*ghorhe*): a wound that in addition to the skin caused damage to its underlying tissue, but it is infectious. This wound include some subgroups as well. In TIM sources, special treatment methods have been mentioned such as dietary plans and using of herbal, mineral and animal drugs, for every type of wounds. On the other hand, the principles mentioned in modern medicine, are considered in TIM too; include, cleaning and washing the wound site from infection and pollutants, using medicines that dry the pus and infections; but it is accented that the applied drugs should not have high drying characteristics but the wound should be wet and its infection and serous fluid should be repelled and allow the meat to grow at the wound. The aim of this study is to review the treatments mentioned in TIM sources for various wounds. Given that the TIM possesses a great potential to cure different diseases, it is possible to arrive to novel achievements in pharmacotherapy using the previous experiences and exploiting today's technology and knowledge.

Chapter 2 - An injury to skin initiates an array of pathophysiological events, including inflammation, tissue remodeling, and tissue repair. However, microbial colonization and invasion of the exposed subcutaneous tissues with pathogenic microorganisms increase the risk of wound infections. The threat is even greater when pyogenic wounds are colonized with antimicrobial resistant pathogens. With almost no new class of antibiotic drugs in the development pipeline, the use of non-antibiotic antibacterial agents, including phytochemicals and metals have extensively been researched to replace or supplement the current arsenal of antimicrobial medications. Furthermore, the application of phages, the natural bacterial predators, has been found to be effective in resolving chronic multi-drug resistant wound infections. Recently, the primary objective of wound management has been revised to address the role of skin microbiome in acute and chronic wound healing. In light of these new paradigms of microbial ecology and beneficial bacterial interactions, probiotics therapy have also emerged as potential pro-healers aiding tissue repair mechanisms associated with skin abrasions. This chapter will discuss in detail the various antibiotic alternative therapies that could be used against antimicrobial resistant bacteria in wound infections.

Chapter 3 - Wound healing is a physiological process that involves several successive and often overlapping phases that lead to the restoration of the integrity of the skin after an injury, accident or surgery: haemostasis and inflammation, proliferation and remodeling. The interruption or slowing down of these processes can cause abnormal or impaired wound healing. There are now numerous data and clinical studies that highlight the role of estrogens on normal cutaneous homeostasis and wound healing. In postmenopausal women, for example, the reduced rate of wound healing processes has been clearly related to estrogen deficiency, especially in relation to inflammation and re-granulation, while treatment with exogenous estrogens can reverse these effects. The authors here the complex role of estrogens and estrogenic derivatives in wound healing process, with a focus on their therapeutic use, and which strategies have been explored to find substances with poor systemic effects.

Chapter 4 - As a complex and highly regulated process occurring in overlapping phases, wound healing is key to retaining physiological function of the skin. Characterised by an excessive and unrelenting inflammatory phase, persistent infection, and diminished cellular response to environmental stimuli, chronic wounds significantly pose a burden to patients and service providers, including the entire healthcare system. Chronic wounds include venous, ischemic and diabetic foot ulcers, and purulent wounds, such as surgical site infections. Most distressing, the response of chronic wounds to exorbitantly expensive conventional therapeutic methods is often diminished, and once healed these wounds are frequently considered "high risk for recurrence", particularly in the case of diabetic foot ulcers. With the projected epidemic of diabetes mellitus and an aging population in developing countries, it is important to substantiate cheaper and safer therapeutic techniques for the management of chronic wounds to allow health care providers access to treatment alternatives for their patients. For this reason, the development of innovative non-invasive therapeutic modalities is crucial. For some time now, photobiomodulation therapy (PBMT), formally referred to as low-level light/laser therapy (LLLT), has been used to induce physiological changes and therapeutic benefits. Despite the overwhelming evidence regarding its therapeutic capability, PBMT is not universally accepted as the induced effects at a tissue, cellular and molecular level are not completely understood, and mistrust or cynicism towards alternative and unconventional medicine. PBMT involves the use of low-powered (usually less than 1 W/cm^2) light emitting diodes (LEDs), lasers or broadband light, mostly in the visible red and near infrared (NIR) light spectrum (600 – 1,100 nm). It is used in a wide variety of applications, and is typically used to alleviate pain, reduce inflammation and oedema, and speed up healing or induce healing in non-responsive chronic wounds of a wide range of aetiologies. Further evidence of the efficiency of existing and future wound therapies is necessitated for their acceptance and appropriate use. This chapter explores the impact of PBMT on wound healing and the basic biochemical reactions involved.

Chapter 5 - Postoperative surgical wound infection (SWI) in the lumbar spine is unfortunately a common and potentially devastating complication. It is associated with increasing morbidity and the need for further surgery. The rate of spinal wound infection in literature ranges from 0.7 to 11.9% . The type of surgery is perhaps the most significant variable affecting the rate of infection. When instrumentation is used for lumbar fusions, the infection rate increases and Staphylococcus aureus is the most common organism causing SWI. Other reported causative organisms include Staphylococcus epidermidis, Enterococcus faecalis, Pseudomonas spp., Enterobacter cloacae and Proteus mirabilis. Gram-negative bacteria are more common in trauma patients. White blood cell count is an unreliable indicator of infection. Erythrocyte sedimentation rate (ESR) may remain elevated for up to six weeks after surgery and C-reactive protein (CRP) levels normalize within two weeks. In regard to the potential role of Procalcitonine (PCT), recent trials demonstrated that PCT may be useful to diagnose neurosurgical patients with SWI. Magnetic resonance imaging (MRI) is the most useful study to diagnose SWI. Gadolinium enhancement improves the diagnostic accuracy of MRI and it should be used whenever an infection is suspected. Rim enhancing fluid collections, ascending epidural collections, the evidence of bone destruction and progressive marrow signal changes are suggestive of infection. The nonoperative treatment of postoperative spinal wound infections is rarely indicated and it is generally limited to significantly immunocompromised patients. Treatment of SWI is centered on the surgical debridement of all necrotic tissue and the obtainment of intra-operative cultures to guide antibiotic therapy. The authors recommend the involvement of an infectious disease specialist to adjust and monitor the efficacy of the antibiotic treatment. In most cases, SWI can be adequately treated while leaving spinal instrumentation in place. For severe SWI, repeat debridements, delayer closure and the involvement of a plastic surgeon may be necessary. In some patients the use of the VAC therapy may be useful for the wound closure. Proven methods to prevent wound infection include prophylactic antibiotics, meticulous adherence to aseptic technique, frequent release of retractors to prevent myonecrosis and shorter operative time.

In: A Closer Look at Wound Infections ...   ISBN: 978-1-53616-816-7
Editor: Joseph E. Keel   © 2020 Nova Science Publishers, Inc.

Chapter 1

TYPES OF WOUND AND WOUND HEALING FROM THE PERSPECTIVE OF TRADITIONAL IRANIAN MEDICINE (TIM)

Maryam Rameshk, PhD*
and Shahram Kalantari Khandani, PhD
Department of traditional pharmacy,
Kerman University of Medical Sciences, Kerman, Iran

ABSTRACT

Wound healing is a complex cascade of events that led to reconstruct a damaged tissue with cellular and biological mechanisms. Along with chemical drugs, in some case, herbal remedies work better and with fewer side effects. Almost 30% of traditional drugs applied to dermal disturbance and wound, while, only 1-3% of modern drugs are allocated to this goal. Traditional Iranian Medicine (TIM) is a rich knowledge source based on herbal drugs for treating diseases including treatment of various wounds. In TIM, wound in general has been known as Tafarrogh-

---

* Corresponding Author's E-mail: mrameshk77@gmail.com.

e-ettesal that means tissue disconnection, which includes different wounds:

Scratch (*kharash*): a superficial wound that cause damage only to the skin.

Wound or injury (*jerahat*): a wound that in addition to the skin caused damage to its underlying tissue, but it is not infectious. In TIM, this type of wound divided into 10 subgroups.

Sore or ulcer (*ghorhe*): a wound that in addition to the skin caused damage to its underlying tissue, but it is infectious. This wound include some subgroups as well.

In TIM sources, special treatment methods have been mentioned such as dietary plans and using of herbal, mineral and animal drugs, for every type of wounds. On the other hand, the principles mentioned in modern medicine, are considered in TIM too; include, cleaning and washing the wound site from infection and pollutants, using medicines that dry the pus and infections; but it is accented that the applied drugs should not have high drying characteristics but the wound should be wet and its infection and serous fluid should be repelled and allow the meat to grow at the wound.

The aim of this study is to review the treatments mentioned in TIM sources for various wounds. Given that the TIM possesses a great potential to cure different diseases, it is possible to arrive to novel achievements in pharmacotherapy using the previous experiences and exploiting today's technology and knowledge.

Keywords: flesh grower, Persian medicine, scratch, Traditional Iranian Medicine, ulcer, wound healing

INTRODUCTION

Since the birth of mankind and for thousands of years, traditional medicine has responded to community health needs. Herbal medicine and the use of herbs and their products for the treatment of various diseases are the main fields of it [1]. Results of studies show that the use of traditional medicine and natural ingredients in the treatment of many diseases and injuries has spread all over the world and more than 80% of the world population use traditional medicine for treatment [2, 3].

Today, due to the adverse effects of chemicals, the use of medicinal plants is on the rise. According to the recommendation of the World Health Organization for the use of medicinal plants, studying the effects of medicinal plants is essential [4].

From the perspective of Iranian Medicine, the basic components of all creatures, including humans, animals, plants, and solids, consisting of four elements, including "fire, air, water and soil." The Iranian school of medicine is based on humoral medicine, meaning that the principles of diagnosis and treatment of diseases are based on the recognition of the four elements mentioned above. Warmth, coldness, wetness, and dryness are the four main properties of each of these elements: fire is hot and dry, the air is warm and wet, the water is cold and wet, and the soil is cold and dry. As a result of the action and reaction of these elements, a uniform quality prevails in the components of the composition called temperament. According to this view, drugs, like other substances, consist of the four elements mentioned and have their own temperament. In fact, drugs affect our body based on the warmth, coldness, wetness and dryness properties [5]. In TIM dating back 10,000 years, treatment and prevention methods for various diseases are divided into three main groups: treatment and prevention with food, treatment and prevention with drugs including herbal, animal, mineral and chemical materials, treatment and prevention with manual interventions including phlebotomy, cupping, dry cupping, massage, surgery, etc. [6]. TIM is a rich source of information on the use of medicinal herbs in the treatment of different diseases, including skin wounds [7]. Almost one-third of traditional remedies are used for skin and wound disorders, while 1–3% of modern remedies are used [8, 9, 10, 11]. Skin wounds are divided into several categories according to their severity and for each, treatment with food, herbal, animal and inorganic drugs are recommended [5, 12, 13, 14]. It should be noted that the discussion of types of wounds and their treatment in TIM is a widespread discussion in this study which briefly examines the types of wounds and their treatment in TIM resources.

METHODS

The traditional medicine books which are used in this chapter:

"Al-Qanun fi al-Tibb"

This book was written by Avicenna (Ibn-e-Sīnā), a Persian physician (Afshana, near Bukhara - Hamadan 980-1037 AD), who was arguably one of the most outstanding medical scientists and practitioners ever, and had a deep influence on medical science. Qanun was the standard text at many medieval universities, including the University of Montpellier and the Catholic University of Leuven, still 1650. It presents a complete system of medicine according to the principles of Galen and Hippocrates (Figure 1).

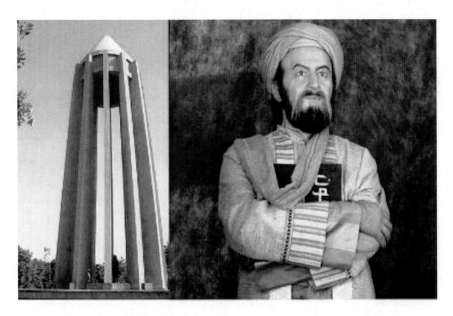

Figure 1. The Tomb of Avicenna, Hamedan, Iran and statue of Avicenna at Milad Tower Fame Museum, Tehran, Iran.

"Zakhireh Kharazmshahi"

In the medical history of Persia another prominent scientist and physician emerges in the early medieval era, who named Jorjani (Zein al-Din Abu Ebrahim Esmail Ebn Jorjani). He was born in Jorjan (Gorgan), a city in the northeast of Iran, in 1042 AD and died in Merv, the capital city of the Seljuk dynasty in 1137 AD. His famous book Zakhireh Kharazmshahi consists of nine books. It is the most important and exhaustive book in medicine and pharmacy written in Persian. The text in this book is simple, fluent and clear, and contains many Persian words (Figure 2).

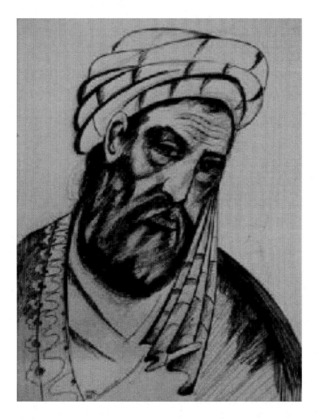

Figure 2. Portrait of Jorjani, by Mrs. Somayeh Tabatabaei (born in 1978). The portrait is kept in the Museum of Shiraz University of Medical Sciences, Shiraz, Iran.

Alabniyeh - an Haqhiqhe al-Adwiya

This book written by Abumansoor Movafagh Ibn Ali Heravi (11th AD) is the first pharmaceutical book in Persian including 29 chapters. It is about herbal medicines and treatment of various diseases.

"Makhzan al Adviyeh"

The largest pharmaceutical manuscript of Persian medicine written by Mohammad Hossein Aghili Khorasani Shirazi in 18th AD; which is one of the latest traditional Persian pharmacopeias containing 28 chapters on natural medicines in alphabetical order involving 1698 monographs.

WOUND DEFINITION FROM THE PERSPECTIVE OF TIM

The wound in TIM sources is known as "Tafarrogh-e-ettesal" meaning Tissue disconnection. It is generally referred to as diseases that cause a rupture in the joints of the organs. The wound is the detachment of the skin and/or the skin and the flesh, whether it is from a cut, a bruise, or a burn, or stick of something in it [5].

There are two types of tissue disconnection causes [5, 12]:

1. External injuries, such as fractures, bruise, and cuts.
2. Internal injuries that are of five types:
    *   A sharp and burning substance that scrape and burns.
    *   The wetness that softens the organ.
    *   The dryness that results in the roughness of the skin.
    *   The accumulation of gas when the gas moves it is pricked.
    *   High humor, which is placed among the organ.

TYPES OF THE WOUNDS IN TIM

Scratch (*kharash*)

A superficial wound that only damaged the skin. In fact, it is a kind of detachment of the skin due to the persecution. This peeling may be without swollen or with swollen, and sometimes the skin itself may be completely detached, cut, or hung. Such as abrasion of the inguinal caused by sweating or sitting on the horse and the abrasion of the heels and toes caused by shoes [5, 12].

Wound or Injury (*jerahat*)

A wound that not only the skin but also the subcutaneous tissue was damaged, but is not purulent, or a wound that causes the skin or flesh and skin to become severed due to cuts, bruises, burns or stick something in it, so that it does not last more than two weeks, or a wound that pure blood seep from it, whether for a long time or short [5].

In Iranian Medicine, injuries are divided into ten types [5, 12]:

1. Straight, smooth, and simple crack that sometimes with no decrease in the flesh.
2. Round and circular wound.
3. Angular and polygonal wound.
4. A wound that has lost some of its flesh.
5. The deep wound but its depth is not clear.
6. The deep wound but its depth is clear.
7. Its flesh is bruised and blood is collected in its components.
8. A wound that has edema.
9. A wound that enters the abdomen and the abdominal muscle is torn and the intestine falls out.
10. A wound that has reached the bone.

Sore or Ulcer (*ghorhe*)

A wound that not only the skin but also the subcutaneous tissue was damaged, but is purulent. The appearance of pus is because the body is unable, waste material enters it, and, on the other hand, because the diseased organ is unable to handle food and digestion, the food becomes waste and pus. If the pus is thick, it is called filth (*vasakh*) , which is pus that is clogged, motionless, and white or black or lees of wine-colored. If the pus is dilute, it is called ichor (*sadid*), which is plasma and composed of dilute and thin humor [5, 12].

In Iranian Medicine, the ulcer is divided into several types:

1- Painful ulcer
2- Pain free ulcer
3- Swollen ulcer
4- No swollen ulcer
5- Clean ulcer
6- Dirty and unclean ulcer (with a lot of humor and moisture attached to it).

In general, the ulcer is either found or seen, or is hidden, and deep.

- A deep ulcer like a hollow tube with a narrow opening is called a fistula (*nāsur*).
- The ulcer that has reached the skin and skin is separated from it, called a poket.
- If the ulcer reaches under the flesh and is loose, it is called a cave.

If the color of the ulcer turns to green and black, it is a bad sign of the ulcer.

TREATMENT IN GENERAL

In any type of wound, the bleeding must first be stopped, but in some cases, it may be expedient to allow a certain amount of blood shed from the wound in order not to swell the wound and not cause fever. It should not be allowed to swell as far as possible because if the wound doesn't swell it will be easily treated, but if swelling or bruising or disintegration occurs in the wound, the blood stays in the wound. This can either cause swelling or festering of the wound. In this case, the wound healing is not possible and swelling should be treated. Therefore, if the bleeding is less than necessary, it should be helped to reach the required bleeding [5].

If a rupture or an ulcer develops in the body, it will improve very quickly if the body has a good temperament, meaning it has less abnormal moisture. If the body has a bad temperament, meaning it is too wet or dry, it may take a long time to heal, especially in the body of those suffering from dropsy or cachexia or leprosy [5].

If the aim is to heal the wound, it must be closed so that both edges of the wound are fully stuck. If the gap is wide and the wound is large, there is a need for triangular pads. The pads should be placed on the wound so that a straight line is found between the two triangular pads, in which case the band is tighter and better placed on the wound than the pads are quadrilateral. The suture is also needed if the slot is full (the flesh is high in it). But if you want the flesh to grow in the wound, it is not necessary to close and only needs to close the wound in two ways:

1. Closing to press the wound to remove pus and dirt from its opening
2. Closing to keep the drug on the wound
   - There should always be somewhere in the wound openings for continuous removal of pus and secretions of the wound.
   - If too much flesh is removed from the wound, it should be used with flesh-grower drugs to compensate for lost flesh [5].

General Topics of Medications Used for Wound Healing

- Medications that remove thorns and arrows: It is a drug with its high absorption that absorbs the thorns and arrows from the depth of body.
- Blood stopping drugs: It is a drug with high contractile properties that stops bleeding.
- Caustic drug: It is a drug that adheres the skin with its burning and drying properties and closes the humor ducts.
- Wound healing drugs: It is the type of drug that adheres two distant edges of the wound. If blood was found during fusion of the two edges of the wound, the drug should be able to rapidly dry the blood present in the wound, and not allow the wound to be infected. Wound healing medication should not be scraper because it is contrary to the physician's goal of treatment. The drug should dry the blood inside the wound so that blood can be used instead of adhesive. If the medication is a scavenger, it eliminates the fake adhesive. Healing drug like flesh-grower do not need to reduce drying power.
- Flesh-grower drug: It coagulates healthy blood and converts it into the flesh. If the drug is too desiccant, it prevents blood from reaching the wound and as a result, there is nothing to convert to the flesh.
- Corrosive medicine: The drug that is needed to eat rotting flesh and inappropriate substances in the wound and must be highly scavenger.
- Terminator and sealant drugs: The sealant drug should be applied to the wound, which should be aligned with the skin when the wound and its flesh are dry [5, 12].

The drug should be administered before the growth of healthy flesh in the wound reaches the level above the skin. Because the final wound healing drug also has a flesh-grower effect, and by applying it to the wound, nature is even more potent and helps. Therefore, any state of the wound condition should be carefully examined. The drug should be used so that when the wound is completely dry, it returns to normal and there is no sign of a wound. Flesh and skin should be in harmony and not seen above or below. If this procedure is not performed well, the sign of wound or ulcer that has healed may remain [5, 12].

It should be noted that plants and animal and mineral substances that affect the treatment of various types of wounds are listed in Tables 1-3.

Recommended Foods for the Treatment of Wounds

At the time of wound healing, the patient should avoid eating blood maker foods such as flesh and sweets. It has been said that if the wound is white, the patient should eat melon and milk, and if it is dark, the patient should eat such things as broad beans, but if the wound is high red, the beef is appropriate but if it is low red lamb is appropriate.

If it is found that the ulcer has bad and contaminated blood, the patient should use a food that produces good blood. If anemia is found to cause ulceration, the patient should use blood maker foods to the blood reach the organs as much as necessary [5, 12].

To fill in the hollow area of the wound that has lost its flesh, you must give the patient a good chymus (producing healthy fluid) because the flesh-grower drug may only promote flesh growth. If its effect is restricted to the growth of the flesh, it can only produce stiff flesh instead of skin that hair does not grow on it [5].

Treatment of Different Types of Wounds

Treatment of Scratch (kharash)

In this case, the separated skin should be stuck in place. You should not cut off the skin as much as possible; the skin should be spread on the first place and glued. This should be repeated several times to make sure that the same cut skin adheres to the first place. If the area where the skin is separated is in sight, it is better to apply the drug after the skin has returned to its place but it should not be closed unless it is not possible. It is better if the medicine is in the open air.

If shedding is light, single and simple medications are sufficient and especially if shedding is on the sole, adhesion of animal lung, and especially lamb lung can result in treatment. If shedding is not associated with swelling, the following medications may be helpful:

1.   Burned old animal skin
2.   Red Zarnikh and oil of *Rosa damascena* locally
3.   Burned Qar' (*Cucurbita pepo* L.) has a strange effect, especially on the shedding of the sole

If the crack is accompanied by shedding, the sealing, welding, and terminator agents and light and astringent medicines such as Aqaqiā (*Acacia arabica*), Balut (*Castanea sativa*), and especially burned Balut is necessary that these light and astringent medicines are sufficient in the treatment of mild shedding, and hidden and invisible shedding.

Sammāq (*Rhus coriaria*) is a very good medication in the treatment of mild shedding and in the treatment of shedding with cracks. Sammāq does not allow for swelling. Spraying remedies to treat shedding pain, and especially if the skin is cracked due to shedding, include: Boiled Adas (*Lens culinaris*), lukewarm seawater spraying on the skin. It is good to put dried lees of wine on the shedding skin. But if the skin is completely separated, you should try to prevent swelling and use drugs that are very dryer and sealing. The cure of a condition where the skin is completely separated is more difficult to shedding.

The cure for absolute scratch, which is just skin erosion, is to bare the area to allow cool air reaches it and spraying cold water and rose water on it and rubbing ice. Spraying burned, milled, and sieved Aqaqiā and Balut as well as boiled or soaked Sammāq are useful. Mordāsanj (Litharge) ground with wine, lukewarm seawater and lees of wine are also useful.

To treat foot abrasion with shoes, it is useful to put a fresh lung, especially lung of the mule. If the lungs are grilled and put on it, it will relieve swelling and pain and will cure it. If it is not swollen, it is useful to burn, grind, and sprinkle old leather shoes, and burned zucchini, oil of *Rosa damascene*, and Zarnikh are also useful [5, 12].

It should be noted that plants and animal and mineral substances that affect the treatment of various types of wounds are listed in Tables 1-3.

Treatment of Any Kinds of Wound or Injury (jerahat)

In some organs, if the wound develops, it can cause severe damage and is dangerous and will most likely cause death unless the wound is very light. These organs include the bladder, kidney, brain, small intestines and liver. But if the heart is injured, death is certain. Those who have an internal wound may die if they get nausea, hiccups, or diarrhea.

If the wound is simple and its flesh is not reduced, it may be sufficient to closing and preventing to reach fat and water to it is sufficient for treatment and not need anything else. Of course, care must be taken that anything like hair and so on does not stick into the cracked layer. The patient should avoid foods and beverages that are blood maker, in order to prevent swelling and healing and no other treatment except closing is required. Other measures to prevent swelling are included moistening a cloth with vinegar and rose water and rubbing it around the wound. Of course, no drug is more beneficial than sour and sweet pomegranates cooked with astringent wine which both prevents swelling and heals wounds [5, 12].

If the wound is round, or the shape is one in which the edges of the wound are apart, or the flesh is separated from it, it should be sutured and not allow to penetrate moist substances. To prevent moisture from entering, drying and inhibiting drugs should be used. If the wound is in the deep, it often closes together by closing and does not need to be exposed and bare. But it is better if it is visible and seen and no harm is done. This disclosure, of course, is necessary when no benefit is achieved from wound closure, especially if the depth of the wound is not affected by bandage and closing and the organ accepts inappropriate substance due to pain and disability caused by the wound [5].

If the wound closure has no effect on the depth of the wound, or the wound is in such a way that there is no way to expel the substance of swelling, or there is a bone at the wound site or the wound becomes fistula and the moisture accumulates excessively. In these cases, it looks like an ulcer, and the wound should be exposed and treated. When exposing the wound, cotton or something like cotton should be put on the wound opening to absorb the moisture that exudes from the wound opening [5].

If the inside of the wound is more wide than the wound opening, it has no choice but to cleave it and it should be cleaved from the side that if the organ moves, the cleft will not open. If the wound is deep, a wick should be smeared with appropriate ointments and oils and put on a wound or it should be put the medicine on the cloth (linen) and close the wound with it. If the tip of the arrow, bone, or thorn is left in the wound and is unavailable, absorbent ointments should first be put on it and then treated. If the swelling becomes severe and materials move to the wound, the opposite organ should be phlebotomy [5].

Some wounds have bad effects, such as a wound in or near the patella, which has very bad consequences and is less likely the patient will survive. If the wound develops in sensitive areas of the muscle and the wound causes seizure and is not curable, the only way to cure it is to cut the muscle. That is, the muscle must be transversely cut and the patient consent to muscle inactivation. But in general, the decision to cut the muscle should be delayed and as much as possible the patient's seizure and anxiety should first be treated [5].

In the case of injuries that are deep, rough, angular, too large or too deep, or has lost the skin with some flesh:

- If the wound is deep and it is in the flesh or it is fresh, the wound dryer should be used.
- In all new injuries, the dryer should be used and the injury should be closed for two to three days until it is firmly closed. After this period, it is best to open the dressing and keep it closed for one or two days.

- If the injury is rough, it is necessary to cleave it and then cure it. If the injury is old, its treatment is like ulcer. If the injury is huge, the member should be cut and separated [12].

- If the injury is deep and the head is tight, it should not be closed so that the pus does not accumulate in the bottom. For this purpose, an old cotton should be placed in the opening to prevent the flesh from growing and, if needed, the old cotton should be smeared with cow oil or olive oil, and then the cloth smeared with the flesh-grower medicines and the required ointments should be placed in the deep of the wound. Each time a smaller cloth should be used to smear with drugs and again put the old cotton smeared with cow oil on its opening until the flesh begins to burst from the depth of the wound and leave no depth left to cause pus. Sometimes the injury should be cleaved so that nothing is left in it that can cause swelling and ulceration after the wound is closed. If it is necessary to cleave the injury, it should be done in the manner will describe [12].

- If the injury is rough and has angles or some flesh has separated along with the skin and the edges of the injury cannot be brought together, it should be stitched in two or three places then put the drug on it and close. The use of moist remedies on the wound should be avoided and inhibitors drugs that prevent the entry of substance into the organ, dryer, and grower should be used. If the flesh of the injury has been bruised and blood has accumulated in the components of dead flesh, it should be undermined as soon as possible with soft medicines. In this type of injury, a moderately potent drying agent should be used because a strong drying agent will cook the food that enters the body and prevent it from turning into flesh, and if the purgative drug is strong, it dilutes the food and destroys the flesh. Therefore, drugs must be moderate in both drying and purging to eliminate excess moisture and convert the remaining blood into flesh. Flesh-grower drugs should have a higher drying effect and no scavenging effect because the purpose is to use a drug (with strong drying effect and no scavenging effect) that will stabilize the blood [12].

- If the injury is in the flesh, the drugs such as leaf of Populus mixed with vinegar or boiled in grape wine, green oak, pomegranate peel, washed Qalimia, dried Lesān ol-hamal (*Plantago major* L.), and washed Shādanaj should be used. Each of these drugs in small injuries results in flesh growth and healing the injury. Along with these drugs, the leaf of Hommāz al-māee (*Rumex aquaticus* L.), leaf of Karm (*Vitis vinifera* L.), leaf of Khas (*Lactuca sativa*), and leaf of Ollaiq (*Rubus fruticosus*) should be used. But if the injury is huge, wet cheese made from sour milk is useful. If the injury is new, the drugs mentioned will suffice. But if the injury is old, Esfidāj with Ās oil (*Myrtus communis* L.) in ointment form, burned Qalqatār, and then boiled with wine, Murr (*Commiphora molmol*) with Qanturiun Saghir extract (*Centaurium min*us), boiled Zaravand mudahraj (*Aristolochia rotunda*) in wine and then crushed, dried, and sieved, dried Lesān ol-hamal (*Plantago major* L.) with Mastaki oil (*Pistacia Lentiscus* L.), or Ās oil (*Myrtus communis* L.) in an ointment form, and the root of Jāvshir (*Opopanax chironium*) mixed with vinegar are useful [12].

It should be noted that plants and animal and mineral substances that affect the treatment of various types of wounds are listed in Tables 1-3.

How to Cleave the Wound

If the wound is in an organ but does not appear and is in the deep and cannot be cured by the drug, the wound must be cleaved to reach the center of the wound. Galen reported some instructions for cleave the wound:

1. For lancing and cleave, the most protuberant, thinnest and narrowest site of wound should be selected.
2. Cleave should be done such that the route of pus flow is downward.

3. When lancing, the situations of skin lines and skin folds should be considered carefully.
4. If the wound is in the groin or armpit, the cleft should accompany the normal skin situation.
5. After cleave, drying drugs without irritant effect should be put on the wound. The resin shell of *Boswellia carterii* is best because it is very astringent.
6. At the time of wound healing, the patient should never come close to the water [5].

Treatment of Various Types of Sore or Ulcer (ghorhe)

General Cure: the food of the patient should be soft. At the beginning of the ulceration or when the ulcer is developing, bathing and bringing hot water to the right position is not good because it absorbs water and increases swelling and makes it harder to heal. Bathing and washing with warm water is not an obstacle when the pain and swelling are reduced and the ulcer festered [5].

If tissue disconnection occurs between the soft organs, three conditions should be considered and treated in three stages:

In the first step, if the separating agent is stable, it must cut off what is flowing to the organ and eliminate any material in the vicinity of the organ.

In the second stage, the cleaved site should be welded with appropriate medications and foods.

In the third stage, as far as possible, it should be prevented from infecting it.

When one of these three stages is resulted, there is no need to try and do the other two steps [5].

Order of treatment for ulcer is as follow:

First, the maturative medications should be used to treat pus. Then polisher drugs should be used to cleanse and then the grower drugs to treat and for the filthy ulcer, the ulcers with high pus, sharp and cleansing medications should be used [12].

The solution to treat the ulcers is to dry them. If the ulcer is pure, it should only be dried. If the ulcer is fetid, corrosive medicines such as Zāj asfar (Yellow vitriol), Zarnikh (orpiment), and Neurah (Quick lime) should be used. If these drugs do not work, the ulcer should be dried with fire. A drug combined with Zangār (Verdigris) and Mum (wax) and oil is useful for purifying and disinfecting the ulcer; the Zangār cleans it and Mum and oil prevent excessive burning [5].

Each ulcer is either simple or compound. If the ulcer is small and simple and not phagedena, two edges of it should be stuck together. However, be careful there are no substances such as oil or dust. The ulcer will heal by this method. If the ulcer is large and the flesh is not reduced, it can still adhere the edges together. If the ulcer is large and it is not possible to adhere the edges, or it is full of pus, or the flesh of the organ is reduced, the only way to cure it is to dry it. If the skin is missing, it has to be sealed. There are two ways to seal it: either by astringent or by a certain amount of Zāj asfar that is useful for drying. If the ulcer is high, and the flesh is missed, as in the deep ulcers, the treatment should not start with sealing, but first with growing the flesh. In addition, it is necessary to examine the main temperament of the organ and ulcer. If the temperament of the organ is very wet and the ulcer secretion is less, a brief drying is sufficient first, as the disease is not very distant from the temperament of the organ. But if the temperament of the organ is dry and temperament of the ulcer is very humid (with high secretion), in the second and third stages it also needs drying to equal the temperament of the organ. In all cases, the condition should be in moderation, which means that the temperament of the body should also be considered, because if the body is very dry and the humidity of the organ is too high, one can consider the state of the body and then dry the ulcer with a mild drug in terms of dryness and wetness. Also, if the body moisture is more than moderate and the body extremity tends to be dry, the same method should be done. The cold temperament ulcer is white and it is calmed by warm medicines. The color of warm temperament ulcer tends to be red and benefits from cold treatments. It may leak something like hot water from the ulcer that burns around it; this may indicate a patient's death. An ulcer that causes hair loss around it is a bad sign. If the ulcer has caused the hair loss around it but the hair is growing again, it means that the ulcer is improving. Drugs that cause flesh to re-growth along with drying should be able to expel pus rather than sealing, welding, and wounds eliminators drugs. Any drug that dries the ulcer without burning is helpful in growing flesh. Round and circular ulcers heal later than other ulcers. Internal ulcers should be treated with a combination of drying, astringent, and penetrative agents, such as honey, which should be combined with drying and astringent medicines. If we want to cure internal ulcer, we have to combine it with astringent and adhesive medications like Tin makhtum. If the blood that reaches the ulcerated organ is bad temperament, something should be done to produce a healthy fluid. If the blood volume is higher than necessary, leading to organ wet, efforts should be made to discharge it, to make the patient's food soft and forced to exercise if possible. If the ulcer causes the bone to become thin and weak and to flow out of the pus, the drug is not the only remedy, but if the bone degeneration is removed by shaving, it should be shaved or cut the bone. The meaning of this sentence is that Ibn Sina means osteomyelitis or bacterial infection of the bone, which is caused by an infectious agent, especially Staphylococcus aureus. Interestingly, today bone sequesters are also removed by sequestrectomy, which is practically the same technique that Ibn Sina has recommended to his students [5].

Treatment of Ulcer That Secrets Plasma

In the treatment of such ulcers, drying and astringent medicines should be used first, followed by the flesh-grower medications that have the scavenging properties. When the temperament is too wet and the effect of drying drug is not clear, it should be enhanced with scavenger drugs like honey and astringent drugs such Shab, Golnar (*Balaustion pulcherrimum*), and its oil and oil of Ās (*Myrtus communis* L.) should be used. It should be noted that some drying drugs have several types, some of which are very cold, such as Afyun (*Papaver sumniferum*) and some very hot, such as Ratinaj (*Cedrus libani*) and some are more temperate such as pomegranate peel, Shab, resin shell of *Boswellia carterii*, Mordāsanj, and Shaqaieq.

Salve that is drying and beneficial: salve made by pummeling fresh walnuts and leaves [5, 12].

Treatment of Filthy Ulcer

Filthy ulcers, which have a lot of pus and secret various moistures, should be treated with scavenger and strong drugs, especially at the beginning of treatment, any drug that is more potent and burner should be used. Then gradually use softer medicines such as Zaravand mudahraj (Aristolochia rotunda) with a little honey and vinegar, root of Sus (*Glycyrrhiza glabra*) with honey, Karasnah (*Vicia ervillia*) flour with sugar candy and Jāvshir (*Opopanax chironium*). Farāsiun (*Lycopus europaeus*) with honey cleanses the ulcer that is purulent.

If the pus is very high, mix the Gandna (*Allium porrum* L.) with honey and place on the ulcer, which is very useful [5, 12].

Treatment of Deep, Cave-Like, and Pocket-Like Ulcers

In the treatment of these three types of ulcers, the ulcer depression should be filled with flesh. This is done by eating foods that produce a lot of blood. From the point of view of drug therapy, the treatment is done with scavenger and drying drugs. First, it should be noted that if the wound is opened and the pus is poured out, it is very good; otherwise, it should be pierced. If piercing is not possible and there is a risk, the wound should be completely cleaved and then treated. If it is not possible to cleave, scavenger and drying drugs should be used as suppository in it. The drug combination should be such that the scavenger and drying drugs do not deactivate each other's effect. Filling the ulcer with the Luf al-kabir (*Dracunculus vulgaris*) has an amazing medicinal effect. In the second grade, Abrun (*Sedum telephium* L.), in the third grade Zanbaq (*Lilium candidum* L.), and in the fourth grade Karasnah flour (*Vicia ervillia*) are useful.

Deep, cave-like, and pocket-like ulcers cannot be cleaned except with fluid and scavenger medicines; honey, seawater, Shab, water ash[1] are a strong and excellent scavenger and washing agents and prevent the material from flowing to it. If the ulcer is swollen, none of these drugs will work. If less pus flows from the ulcer and the underside of the ulcer is

---

[1] Water ash: Water in which ash is poured and boiled several times, then smooth.

relax, one should guess that it sticks. In such a case, due to the strong bonding pressure and strong drug, the internal adhesion may be eliminated and the pus can be and removed, then the ulcer is dried and adhered and the skin based on the flesh [5, 12].

Treatment of Fetid and Bad Ulcers

First, the dominant and bad humor should be removed from the body and the temperament of the entire body and its organs should be corrected, and if necessary, cupping and leech should be used to remove bad blood. If the fetid ulcer becomes excessively rancid, it may need to be cauterized by fire or may require the use of a hot temperament drug. In many cases, infectious ulcers should be removed by sharp and trenchant drugs or iron tool so that smooth blood and clean flesh or white bones appear. The pain caused by sharp medications can be reduced with cow's oil so that they are refreshed every hour. No hot swelling should be allowed in the ulcer.

If the ulcer cannot be cured, the ulcerated organ must be cut off so that the human body gets rid of the stench of ulcer. The treatment of all infectious wounds is to clean the pus and infection, as noted in the treatment of filthy ulcer. It can be treated by washing with seawater and applying for the mentioned medicines, then growing the flesh locally using drugs that have a mild drying and scavenging effect, such as Kondor (*Boswellia carterii*), Barley flour, Karasnah flour (*Vicia ervillia*), root of Susan (*Iris florentina* L.) and the like. After the flesh has grown and the surface has been smoothed, it is necessary to treat the ulcer. If the surface of the spot is not smooth and it is damp and septic, stronger drying drugs and honey should be used. If the dryness is too high, the surface of the ulcer is always moist and deep, and its edges become stiff and red, in this case you should use ointment that has a higher oil phase. Each drug used should be placed on the spot for three days [5, 12].

Treatment of Wormy Ulcer

If the wet ulcer becomes infectious, septic and wormy, it should be treated with drying agents, such as the Tin makhtum ground with vinegar, which must of course be washed with wine first. Medications that kill the worm and prevent its reappearance include decoction of Afsantin (*Artemisia absinthium* L.), decoction of Qanturiun saghir (*Centaurium minus*), or decoction of Farāsiun (*Lycopus europaeus*). The ulcer is first washed with these decoctions, and then Afsantin, Qanturiun saghir, and the Farāsiun are ground and mixed with salt and sprinkled on locality. It is better if the powder is moistened with wine [5, 12].

Treatment of Balkhi Ulcer

This type of ulcer most commonly occurs in the Balkh region (one of the cities of ancient Iran which is now one of Afghanistan's cities near Mazar-e-Sharif) called balkhi ulcer. This type of ulcer does not exceed the surface of the flesh, it is accompanied by a heartbeat and may cause fainting and can occur with or without fever. Phlebotomy should be performed first for treatment, and the patient should use every morning juice and sour syrups and tablets of Kāfur (*Cinnamomum camphora*) and temperate foods that tend to be cold and wet. It is very useful if the patient is exposed to cool air [12].

Treatment of Corrosive Ulcer without Infection

The treatment is similar to the treatment of balkhi ulcers. Use of leeches to remove bad material and in many cases it is necessary to remove the ulcer with a clean iron tool, or to separate the member from the body so as not to corrupt the other members. If the corrosive ulcer has no infection and heat and is not hot temperament, spraying cold water, Ās water, Rose water, and astringent wine is useful. If the uninfected corrosive ulcer is hot, the vinegar mixed with Rose water and the like from cold water should be sprayed on the ulcer. Also, salves derived from pomegranate peel, lentil, and the fresh leaf of Ās or leaf of Hommāz al-māee is useful. Putting Tin rumi with vinegar, burnt dried pumpkin, green leaf of olive tree on the ulcer is useful [5, 12].

Treatment of the Ulcer That Has Become a Fistulous Ulcer

Treatment of new fistulous ulcer is easier than the older one, especially if it is hollow, in which case there is no choice but to scrape around it with an iron tool, wipe it, or cauterize by fire or burn with sharp medicine, which is painful, especially if they are close to a major organ such as the heart and liver. Generally, the edges of fistulous ulcer should be scraped with an iron tool, and the rotten flesh should be removed and if it is hollow, it should be cleaved and then cauterize and then treated with salve and burning with a sharp and trenchant drug. Burning with a sharp and trenchant drug is done to burn rotten flesh so that it can be separated and removed [12].

Treatment of the Ulcers That Corrupt the Bone

In many cases, the ulcer becomes old and fetid, and the infection reaches the bone. If the infection does not reach the bone, it should be scrapped, but if the bone and marrow are corrupted it should be cut off. If the arm bone or leg bone is corrupted and close to the joint, the joint should be opened and the bone brought out. If the thoracic vertebrae become rotten, cutting it is dangerous due to the spinal cord, but some physicians cauterize the rotten bones to collapse. If a small bone was present in the injuries and ulcers, it should not be brought out; it should be given back to the nature of the body, and then help the nature of the body to eject it. It should not be moved by hand or medicine until it is ejected by the nature of the body and brought close to the skin. Then the drugs that bring out the bone should be used because if it is moved before it is ejected, it may cause seizures and severe fever and the ulcer can become a fistulous ulcer. Some of the drugs that bring out the bone are Oshaq (*Dorema ammoniacum*) and Moql (*Commiphora mukul*) which should be ground with Susan oil and use as salve [12].

Treatment of Ulcers Those Are Difficult to Heal

It includes ulcers that are extremely corrupt and far from healing. Seven causes make recovery difficult:

- High blood volume; in this case first need phlebotomy and purgation then ulcer treatment

-   Anemia; In this case, the whole body, ulcer, and around it become dry and thin, first the anemia must be resolved and then warmed with warm water until the member becomes red and softens around the ulcer. In many cases, it is useful to put a humid cloth with warm water on the ulcer. Black salve is also useful.

Black salve: Beeswax, olive oil, Elk (*Pistacia terebinthus*), and Zeft (*Cedrus libani*) are equally mixed by heat.

-   Poor blood quality that is in two ways: Bad moisture may be mixed with the blood and increase the moisture content in the ulcer and its laxity. Another is that a sharp and burning humor mixed with blood; treatment after evacuation is the treatment of the filthy ulcer already mentioned. Generally, sharp and drying medications should be used to dry the ulcer, then use cow oil to eliminate rotten flesh and then use flesh-grower drugs, sometimes cauterize the ulcer is useful. If the cause of the bad blood is sharp and burning humor mixed with it, its treatment is after evacuation, removing the bad blood by cupping and then using drying medicines for treatment.
-   If some type of dystemperament prevails over the whole body and over that member; temperament correction must be done.
-   The presence of edema in a member that is above the ulcer and the substance of the edema enters the ulcer, for example, if there is an edema in the liver and spleen and an ulcer is formed on the leg, the ulcer will not heal until the edema of liver or spleen removes.
-   Bad or stiff flesh on or below the ulcer; first it should be wound with an iron tool to allow blood to flow out, then remove the stiff flesh and then treat it.
-   Bone in the ulcer; first it should be bared and shaved to be cleaned or cut it off if possible [5, 12].

It should be noted that plants and animal and mineral substances that affect the treatment of various types of wounds are listed in Tables 1-3.

Table 1. The plants using in TIM for wound healing [5, 12-14]

Family	Scientific name	Traditional name	Part used	Application	Therapeutic effect
Adoxaceae	*Sambucus nigra* L.	Khamān kabir	Leaf	Plaster	-fresh leaf: Wound healing
Alliaceae	*Allium porrum*	Herbah	Leaf	Plaster	-Wound healing
Amaranthaceae	*Amaranthus graecizans* L.	Baqlat al – yamaniyat, Sefid marz	Root	Topical	-Treatment of secretory ulcer
	Amaranthus blitum L.				
	Beta vulgaris	Selq	Root, leaf	Plaster	- Complete treatment of filthy ulcer
	Allium Akaka	Kurrāth	Leaf	Plaster	- Treatment of filthy ulcer
Amaryllidaceae	*Narcissus tazetta*	Narjes	-Bulb, Flower	-Powder, Plaster	-Treatment of large wound -Wound healing - Blood stopper - Ulcer cleaner - Thorn and arrow absorber from the body depth
			-Bulb	-Oral	- Wound healing
			-Oil	-Liniment	- Wound healing
	Allium ascalonicum L.	Osqordiun	Bulb	Plaster	- Treatment of large wound and filthy ulcer
	Allium sativum L.	Thum	Bulb	Plaster	- Treatment of intractable ulcer
Anacardiaceae	*Pistacia atlantica*	Botm, Bane, Habbah al-khadra	-Gum	-Plaster	-Wound cleaner - Wound pus dryer -Flesh grower
	Pistacia Lentiscus L.	Mastaki	-Seed	- Plaster -Powder	- Rigid wounds softener -Treatment of ulcer and flesh grower

Table 1. (Continued)

Family	Scientific name	Traditional name	Part used	Application	Therapeutic effect
Anacardiacea	Rhus coriaria	Sammāq	-Leaf	-Extract, Decoction	-Flesh grower
			-Shell of Seed	-Plaster, Liniment	- Treatment of filthy ulcer - Prevents the spread of filthy ulcer
			-Extract of leaf, branch and wood, decoction of shell of seed with leaf, branch and wood	-Liniment	- Treatment of wet ulcer
			-Extract of cooked leaf	- Liniment	- Treatment of intractable ulcer
			-Gum	-Liniment, Plaster	- Wound healing, treatment of filthy ulcer, prevents the spread of filthy ulcer
	Dorema ammoniacum	Oshaq	Oleo-gum-resin	Plaster	- Filthy ulcer healing - Destroyer of rotten flesh
Apiaceae	Opopanax chironium	Jāvshir, Gāvshir	-Root	Plaster	- Treatment of chronic ulcer
			-Bloom	Plaster	- Treatment of wound
			-Whole plant	Plaster	- Treatment of filthy ulcer
	Daucus carota	Jazar, Gazar	Leaf, Seed	Plaster	- Treatment of corrosive ulcer
	Cuminun cyminum L.	Cammun	Seed	Powder	-Wound healing
	Apium graveolens	Karafs, Karasb	Leaf	Plaster	- Wound healing
	Ferula gummosa	Bārzad, Qennah	Gum resin	Plaster	- Destroyer of rotten flesh

Family	Scientific name	Traditional name	Part used	Application	Therapeutic effect
	Anethum graveolens	Shebet	Seed	Powder	- Ash: wet and filthy ulcer dryer - Treatment of loose ulcer
	Ferula asafetida	Anjodān	Seed, Root	Plaster	-Wound healing
	Ferula persica	Sakbinaj	Gum	Plaster	-Wound healing
Apiaceae	*Peucedanum officinale* L.	Bakhur ol-akrād	Root	Powder	- Treatment and wound intractable dryer
	Eryngium caeruleum	Qarasa'na	Root	-Oral - Plaster	-Decoction: edema reducer and wound remover - Dissolution of edema and wet ulcer
	Coriandrum sativum L.	Kozborah	-Leef, Branch -Seed	- Plaster - Powder	- Treatment of ulcer -Blood stopper
	Cynanchum vincetoxicum	Qunna barā	Leef	Plaster	- Treatment of filthy ulcer of breast
Apocynaceae	*Holarrhena antidysenterica*	Tivāj	Bark	Fume	-Blood stopper
	Calotropis Procera	Kharak, Oshar	-Leef -Fibers inside of fruit	-Powder - Plaster	- Prevents the spread of cancerous ulcer - Filthy ulcer cleaner, ulcer dryer - Destroyer of waste and rotten flesh -Fresh fibers: blood stopper, flesh grower
Aquifoliaceae	*Ilex aquifolium* L.	Jidār	Leef	Powder	- Wound healing
Araceae	*Dracunculus vulgaris*	Luf, luf al-kabir Luf al-hayyah	-Leaf, Spathe, Fruit, Root	Plaster, Solution	- Treatment of fresh and wet wound, fistula and filthy ulcer -Flesh grower, infectious wound cleaner -Leaf: wound healing
	Arum italicum L.	Luf al-jud, luf al-saghir	- Root	-Liniment	- Destroyer of waste flesh and flesh grower - Treatment and wound dryer - Treatment of cancerous ulcer

Table 1. (Continued)

Family	Scientific name	Traditional name	Part used	Application	Therapeutic effect
Araliaceae	*Hedera helix*	Lablāb kabir	-Leaf	-Plaster	- Treatment of large wound
		Shahmieh (black type)	-Leaf	-Plaster	-Fresh leaf: wound healing -Dry leaf: dryer and destroyer of cancerous ulcer
Arecaceae	*Phoenix dactylifera* L.	Tamr	-Core -Unripe date	-Powder - Plaster - Plaster	-Burnt: Treatment of filthy ulcer - healing of fresh wound - Healing of fresh wound
Aristolochiaceae	*Aristolochia indica* *Aristolochia rotunda*	Zarāvand tawil Zaravand mudahraj	Root	Plaster	- Treatment of ulcer -Flesh grower - Filthy ulcer cleaner - Thorn and arrow absorber from the body depth
Asparagaceae	*Urginea scilla steinh.*	Squill, Onsol	Bulb	Plaster	- Ulcer dryer
Asparagaceae	*Muscari comosum*	Balbus, Basal ol-ziz	Bulb	Plaster	- Treatment of secretory ulcer - Scar removal - Black spots remover caused by the wound
Asparagaceae	*Dracaena cinnabari*	Dam ol-akhawain	Sap	-Oral, Plaster -Powder	- Ulcer and fresh wound healing -Blood stopper and wound healing - Treatment of different types of wounds -Flesh grower

Family	Scientific name	Traditional name	Part used	Application	Therapeutic effect
Asphodelaceae	Aloe littoralis	Sebr	Sap	Plaster, powder	- Treatment of filthy and intractable ulcer and fresh wound - Dryer and wound healing
	Asphodelus ramosus L.	Khunthā	Root	Plaster	- Treatment of filthy and intractable ulcer
	Chrysanthemum partenium L.	Oqhown	-Whole plant -Oil	-Plaster - Liniment	- Healing of fistula, intractable and filthy ulcer - Treatment of muscle wound
	Tragopogon pratensis L.	Lahyat al-tais	-Leaf, Flower - Flower	-Powder -Liniment	- Wound healing and treatment of old ulcers and removing the infection -Extract of flower: removes the wound infection
Asteraceae	Centaurea cyanus L.	Qanturiun	Leaf, Flower	Plaster	- Fresh wound healing - Fistula and fresh, old and deep wound sealing and healing
	Centaurea Centaurium L.	Qanturiun kabir	Root	Plaster	-Fresh or dry root: effective in healing of fresh, old and deep wound
	Carlina gummifera	Khāmālaun	Root	Plaster	- Treatment of malignant and corrosive ulcer
	Lactuca sativa	Khas	Leaf	Powder	-Burnt: wound healing
	Chondrilla juncea L.	Khandarili	Gum	Liniment	- Destroyer of waste flesh
	Cirsium rhizocephalum	Dhanab al-sabo'a	Arial part	Plaster	- Wound healing
	Achillea millefolium	Satratiotos	Arial part	Powder	-Blood stopper and treatment of old and fresh wound
	Senecio vulgaris L.	Irifāron, Irighāron	Whole plant	Plaster	-Wound healing

Table 1. (Continued)

Family	Scientific name	Traditional name	Part used	Application	Therapeutic effect
	Inula viscosa	Tobāqa, Tayyun	-Leaf -Oil	- Plaster - Liniment	- Wound healing without causing pus - Blood stopper - Wound healing
Asteraceae	*Saussurea lappa*	Qost	Root	Powder	-Old root: Treatment of wet ulcer
	Onopordum acanthium	Shokāee	Root, Seed	Plaster	- Wound healing
	Artemisia vulgaris L.	Brenjāsaf	Whole plant	Powder	-Burnt: ulcer dryer
	Artemisia santolina	Qaisum	Flower	Plaster	-Dissolvent of edema and wound healing
Athyriaceae	*Athyrium filix femina*	Sarakhs	Root	Powder	- Treatment of wet and intractable wound
Berberidaceae	*Berberis Aristata*	Dārahald	Wood	Plaster, Oral	- Treatment of wound and ulcer
Boraginaceae	*Alkanna tinctoria*	Havāchoobe, Abokhalsā, Khas al-hemār	Root	-Plaster - Liniment	- Treatment of filthy and old ulcer - Wound healing
	Cynoglossum officinale	Lesān al-kalb	Leaf	Plaster	- Wound healing, treatment of fresh wound -Flesh grower in old ulcer
	Eruca sativa	Jerjir, Taretizak	Leaf	Plaster	- Scar removal
	Brassica oleracea	Karnab, Kornob	Leaf	Plaster	-Wound healing - Treatment of deep wound - Prevents the spread of ulcer
Brassicaceae	*Morettia canescens* Boiss.	Hum al-majus	Flower	Powder	- Blood stopper
	Raphanus sativus L.	Fujl	-Root -Seed	-Plaster -Plaster - liniment	- Treatment of filthy and cancerous ulcer - Treatment of gangrene ulcer - Black and green spots remover caused by the wound

Family	Scientific name	Traditional name	Part used	Application	Therapeutic effect
Brassicaceae	*Genus Alyssum*	Tudari	Leaf, Seed	Plaster	- Treatment of ulcer -Fresh leaf: prevents corruption of fresh wound
	Commiphora opobalsamum L.	Balasān	Oil	Oral, Plaster, liniment	- Ulcer cleaner
Burseraceae	*Boswellia carterii* *Boswellia serrata*	Kondor	-Resin	-Powder, Plaster	- Scar removal - Treatment of deep fresh wound -Prevents the spread of ulcer -Wound healing and flesh grower
			-Shell of resin	-Powder, Plaster	-Treatment of fresh wound and scar removal - Prevents the spread of ulcer and ulcer cleaner - Flesh grower and wound dryer - Correction of old wound and ulcer
				-Fume	- Ulcer cleaner and flesh grower
	Commiphora molmol	Murr	Gum	Plaster, Powder, liniment	- Treatment of filthy ulcer - Flesh grower - Scar removal -Wound healing - Wound and ulcer dryer and prevents wound infection
	Icica icicariba DC.	Lāmi	Oleoresin	Powder, liniment	- Healing of large wound

Table 1. (Continued)

Family	Scientific name	Traditional name	Part used	Application	Therapeutic effect
Cactaceae	Opuntia ficus-indica Opuntia humifusa	Raqah yamāni, Raqā'	Leaf	Plaster	-Wound healing
Calophyllaceae	Mesua ferrea	Nāmushk	Bloom	Plaster	- Ulcer dryer
	Papaver sumniferum	Afyun	Sap	Plaster	- Ulcer and wound dryer
Canabinaceae	Cannabis Sativa L.	Qennab	Leaf	Powder	- Corroded leaf: treatment and wet wound and ulcer dryer
Capparidaceae	Capparis spinosa L.	Kabar, Kurak	-Bark of root	-Plaster -Powder	- Healing and treatment of filthy ulcer - Destroyer of waste flesh
			-Leaf	- Plaster	-Fresh leaf: siccative and treatment of filthy ulcer -Dry leaf: old wound dryer
			-Fruit	- Plaster	-Fresh fruit: siccative and treatment of filthy and cancerous ulcer
Caprifoliaceae	Nardostachys Jatamansi	Sonbol	Root, Leaf	Powder, Plaster	-Wound healing - Ulcer dryer
Caryophyllaceae	Acanthophyllum squarroum	Āzarbu, Artanithā	Root	Powder	- Treatment of filthy ulcer
	Holosteum umbellatum L.	Jabarah	Whole plant	Drop	- Broth: wound healing
Chenopodiaceae	Salsola Salicornia	Ushnān	Whole plant	Liniment	-Ash: Destroyer of waste flesh
	Camphorosma monspeliaca	Raihān al-kāfur	-Juice -Whole plant	-Oral - Powder	-Blood stopper - Treatment of wound and ulcer

Family	Scientific name	Traditional name	Part used	Application	Therapeutic effect
Cistaceae	Cistus creticus	Lādhan	Resin	Liniment	-Treatment of old and intractable wound - Destroyer of rotten flesh
Colchicaceae	Colchicum speciosum	Suranjān	Bulb	Powder	- Treatment of old ulcer
Convolvulaceae	Convolvulus scammonia	Saqmuniā	Sap of root	Plaster	-Wound healing
	Calystegia sepium L.	Lablāb, Qissus		Plaster	- Scar removal and prevents the spread of ulcer - Treatment of filthy ulcer and different types of wounds
	Cressa cretica L.	Anthalis	Whole plant	Powder	- Treatment of ulcer and wound
	Convolvulus hystrix	Zari'a	Arial part	Fume	- Effective in wound healing quickly
Crassulacea	Sedum telephium L.	Abrun	Leaf, Flower	Plaster	- Treatment of filthy ulcer and old wound
	Cotyledon umbilicus L.	qutulidon	Leaf, Root	Plaster	-Extract: wound edema reducer
Cucurbitaceae	Bryonia alba L.	Fāsharā	-Root	-Plaster	- Black spots and scar remover caused by the wound, treatment of cancerous ulcer - Destroyer of rotten flesh
Cucurbitaceae	Cucurbita pepo L.	Qar'	-Fruit, Leaf Bark	-Plaster Powder	-Pus cleaner -Burnt: blood stopper
Cupressaceae	Juniperus Sabina L.	Abhol, Avers	Fruit, Leaf	-Powder - Plaster	-Powder of fruit: treatment of wound and infectious ulcer - Plaster of fruit: Prevents the spread of ulcer - Plaster of leaf: removal of red stain resulted from wound

Table 1. (Continued)

Family	Scientific name	Traditional name	Part used	Application	Therapeutic effect
Cupressaceae	*Cupressus sempervirens*	Sarw	Leaf, Branch, Fruit	Powder, Plaster	-Fresh leaf, branch and fruit: treatment of wet ulcer and fresh wound -Burnt leaf: treatment of wet and fresh wound and ulcer -Cooked leaf (Plaster): blood stopper, treatment and wound dryer Fruit: treatment of wet ulcer and wound dryer Juice of fruit: treatment of ulcer and filthy ulcer cleaner
	Tetraclinis articulata	Sandarus	Gum	Powder	- Wound healing
Cyperaceae	*Cyperus papyrus*	Bardi, Papyrus, Qertās	-Root	-Powder	Burnt root: treatment of wet wound, treatment of fresh and old wound, treatment of intractable ulcer and blood stopper of fresh wound
			-Bark of stem	-Powder -Topical	- Wet filthy and non-filthy ulcer dryer, treatment and dryer of foot wound caused by shoes - Flesh grower when the injured organ is wrapped in it
	Cyperus rotundus	So'ad	Root	Powder	-Flesh grower in wet chronic wound

Family	Scientific name	Traditional name	Part used	Application	Therapeutic effect
Dipterocarpaceae	*Shorea robusta* Roth.	Qaiqahan, Qaiqahar	Gum	Liniment, Plaster	- Scar removal, treatment of fistula, fresh and old wound and ulcer - Treatment of chronic and deep wound and ulcer
	Vateria indica	Kahrobā	Resin	Powder	- Blood stopper and wound healing
Ebenaceae	*Diospyros ebenum*	Ābnus	Wood chips	-Powder	-Blood stopper of fresh wound, wound healing and treatment of old wound -Burnt and washed filing: treatment of chronic ulcer
				- Liniment	- Filthy ulcer dryer -Flesh grower
Elaeagnaceae	*Elaeagnus angustifolia*	Ghubairā	Leaf	Plaster	-Fresh and dry: pus cleaner and treatment of wound and ulcer
Equisetaceae	*Equisetum arvense*	Dhanab al-khail, Amsukh	Arial part	-Plaster -Powder	-Treatment of large and cancerous wound -Blood stopper and flesh grower
	Ricinus communis	Kherva'	Oil	Liniment	- Treatment of wet ulcer
	Jatropha curcas L.	Bak rindeh	Sap	Liniment	-Wound healing -Blood stopper
Euphorbiaceae	*Euphorbia resinifera*	Afarbiun, Farbiun	Gum	Liniment	- Destroyer of waste flesh
	Euphorbia antiquorum L.	Zaqqum	Leaf, Flower	Plaster	-Fresh leaf or flower : Treatment of fresh wound
	Mallotus philippinensis	Qenbil	Seed	Powder	- Wound healing - Wet ulcer dryer

Table 1. (Continued)

Family	Scientific name	Traditional name	Part used	Application	Therapeutic effect
	Vicia faba	Bāqelā	Seed	Plaster	- Treatment of muscle ulcer - Rigid wounds softener
	Calicotome spinose	Darshisha'ān, Ghendol	Bark	Plaster	- Wound healing
	Cicer arietinum	Hemmas	Seed	Powder	- Healing of filthy ulcer
	Lotus corniculatus	Handagugi	Leaf, Seed	Juice	- Treatment of filthy ulcer
	Trigonella foenum Graecum	Holbe	Leaf, Seed	Plaster	- Scar removal - Treatment of ulcer
	Anthyllis vulneraria	Anthalis	Whole plant	Powder	- Wound pain Reduction - Treatment of ulcer and wound
Fabaceae	*Vicia ervillia*	Karasnah	Seed	- Liniment - Plaster	- Scar removal and deep wound healing and filthy ulcer cleaner - Prevents the spread of ulcer, cancerous ulcer remover and flesh grower
	Indigofera tinctoria	Nil	Extract	Plaster	- Treatment of filthy and cancerous ulcer - Wound healing and treatment of old wound and ulcer - Thorn and arrow absorber from the body depth
	Glycyrrhiza glabra	Sus, Mahak	Extract	Plaster	- Wound healing
	Lens culinaris	Adas	Seed	Plaster	- Treatment and filthy ulcer cleaner - Filling of deep wound with flesh - Blood stopper

Family	Scientific name	Traditional name	Part used	Application	Therapeutic effect
	Acacia Arabica	Aqaqiā, Shaukah misriya, Umm ghilān, Qarz	-Root, Seed -Leaf -Fruit - Bark of stem and branch	-Plaster -Plaster -Plaster -Plaster	- Treatment of wound - Fresh leaf: flesh grower and treatment of wet and large wound - Treatment of large wound - Blood stopper of fresh wound
	Lupinus angustifolius L.	Tormes	Seed	Plaster	- Treatment of filthy ulcer -Effective for hard wound
	Astragalus fasciculifolius	Anzarut	Gum	Plaster	- Pus cleaner and wound and ulcer dryer - Destroyer of waste flesh - Flesh grower and wound healing - Blood stopper
Fabaceae	*Caesalpinia sappan* L.	Baqam	Arial part	Powder	- Treatment of old ulcer and fresh wound - Blood stopper - Ulcer dryer
	Tamarindus indica	Tamr hindi	Bark	Powder	- Treatment of ulcer and wound
	Dorycnium sp.	Dārufinon	Arial part	Powder	- Blood stopper - Wound healing
	Cassia acutifolia	Sanā makki	Leaf	Plaster	- Treatment of old wound - Treatment of intractable ulcer and wound healing
	Acacia catechu	Kāt	Gum	Powder, Liniment	- Hot wound dryer
	Astragalus gummifer	Kathirā	Gum	Plaster	- Treatment of hot and cold wound
	Lathyrus sativus L.	Khollar, Jalbān	Seed	Plaster	-Flesh grower

Table 1. (Continued)

Family	Scientific name	Traditional name	Part used	Application	Therapeutic effect
Fagaceae	*Castanea sativa*	Balut	Fruit, Leaf, Avellana	-Plaster	- Wound healing -Leaf: treatment of fresh and wet wound -Ash: blood stopper -Burnt and fresh fruit: prevents the spread of ulcer
				-Plaster, Oral	- Avellana: powerful wound dryer, blood stopper and wound healing
	Gentiana lutea	Jentianā	Root	Plaster	- Treatment of intractable wound and ulcer
Gentianaceae	*Centaurium minus*	Qanturiun saghir	Fruit, Leaf, Stem	Plaster	- Fresh fruit, leaf or stem: effective in healing and sealing of large fresh, old and intractable wound -Dry fruit, leaf or stem: deep cancerous ulcer dryer, prevents large fresh and old wounds rupture, wound healing and edema reducer
Haloragaceae	*Myriophyllum spicatum* L.	Hozonbul	Root	Plaster	-Fresh and dry: wound healing
Hypericaceae	*Hypereium perforatum* L.	Heufariqun	Leaf	-Plaster	- Healing of large wound - Treatment and cleaner of filthy ulcer and large wound - Wet wound dryer
				-Powder	- Treatment and cleaner of loose and filthy ulcer

Family	Scientific name	Traditional name	Part used	Application	Therapeutic effect
Iridaceae	Iris florentina L.	Irsa, Susan	-Root	-Plaster	-Treatment of filthy ulcer, healing of fistula and flesh grower - Pus cleaner and wound healing
			-Extract of root -Decoction of root -Leaf and flower	-Liniment - Liniment - Liniment - Plaster	- Treatment of wet wound - Treatment of wound around the muscles - Treatment of wound and chronic ulcer -Wound healing
	Crocus sativus L.	Za'farān	- Oil of stamen -Leaf	- Liniment -Plaster	- Cleaning of intractable ulcer - Treatment of fresh wound - Filthy wound cleaner
Juglandaceae	Guglans regia	Jowz, Gowz	-Gum - Hard shell of fruit	-Plaster - Powder	- Treatment of ulcer - Wound dryer
	Melissa offisinalis	Bādranjboyah	Flower, Leaf	Topical	- Treatment of ulcer
	Teucrium scordium	Jo'adah, Anbar bid	Arial part	Plaster	-Fresh plant: treatment of wet wound -Dry plant: treatment of filthy ulcer - Healing of large wound
Labiatae	Ajuga chamaepitys (L.) Schreb	Kamāfitus	Leaf	Plaster	-Cleaning of chronic ulcer and filthy ulcer, treatment of wound and large filthy ulcer -Fresh wound healing
	Teucrium chamaedrys	Kamāzarius	Arial part (leaf, seed, flower)	Plaster	- Treatment of filthy and chronic ulcer
	Lamium purpureum L.	Alusis, Palihim	Leaf, Branch	Plaster	- Treatment of filthy ulcer

Table 1. (Continued)

Family	Scientific name	Traditional name	Part used	Application	Therapeutic effect
	Ocimum gratissimum	Raihān sulaimāni	Arial part	Plaster	- Prevents the spread of ulcer
	Lavandula vera, Lavandula officinalis	Khazāmi, Shab bou	Flower	Plaster	- Wound healing - Edema reducer
	Thymus vulgaris L.	Sa'atar, Āvishan	Leaf	Plaster	- Treatment of wound
Labiatae	*Lycopus europaeus, Marrubium vulgare* L.	Farāsiun	Leaf	Plaster	- Wound edema reducer -Pus cleaner - Treatment of old, infectious and filthy ulcer - Destroyer of rotten flesh
	Origanum maru L.	Marw, Marmāhur	Seed	Plaster	-Pus cleaner
	Salvia officinalis L.	Lesān al-ebel	Leaf	Powder	- Wound healing - Ulcer dryer - Cancerous ulcer cleaner
	Cinnamomum zeylanicum	Dārsini	Bark	Plaster	- Treatment of ulcer
	Cinnamomum cassia	Salikhea	Bark	Plaster	- Treatment of soft ulcer
Lauraceae	*Cinnamomum camphora*	Kāfur	Gum	Powder	- Treatment of cancerous ulcer and hot wound - Treatment of fresh wound -Blood stopper and reduce wound pain
Leguminosae	*Melilotus officinalis Trigonella grandiflora*	Eklil ol-malek	Fruit	Plaster	- Rinses secretory wound and ulcer
Liliaceae	*Allium cepa*	Basal	Bulb	Plaster	- Treatment of filthy ulcer - Treatment of flaky feet
	Allium porrum L.	Gandna	Leaf	Plaster	- Treatment of wound and blood stopper

Family	Scientific name	Traditional name	Part used	Application	Therapeutic effect
Liliaceae	*Allium sativum* L.	Sum	Bulb	Plaster	- Treatment of large wound
	Eremurus persicus	Eshrās, Serish	Root	Plaster	- Treatment of wound and filthy ulcer
	Lilium candidum L.	Zanbaq	Bulb	Powder, Plaster	-Treatment of large wound -Wound healing - Blood stopper - Ulcer cleaner - Thorn and arrow absorber from the body depth
Linaceae	*Linum usitatissimum* L.	Kattān	-Bark	-Powder	-Blood stopper and wound dryer and wound healing
			-Seed	- Plaster	- Wound healing and reduce wound pain
				-Powder	-Burnt: wound dryer and reduce wound pain
				-Oil	- Wound healing and reduce wound pain
Loranthaceae	*Loranthus europaeus*	Debq	Berrie	Juice	- Treatment of old and filthy ulcer - Intractable wound and edema remover
Lytheraceae	*Lawsonia inermis*	Henna	Leaf	Powder, Plaster	- Ulcer and fresh wound healing
	Abutilon theophrasti Medic.	Abutilon	Leaf	Plaster	- Healing wet and fresh wound
Malvaceae	*Gossypium herbaceum* L.	Qoton	Cotton	- Plaster	-Burnt: dryer and pus absorber from the deep ulcers depth
				- Powder	- Burnt: wounds destroyer and dryer - Destroyer of waste rotten flesh from the old wounds and pus absorber from the depth of them

Table 1. (Continued)

Family	Scientific name	Traditional name	Part used	Application	Therapeutic effect
Meliaceae	*Azadirachta indica*	Nim	-Leaf	-Extract - Plaster	-Wound healing - Cancerous ulcer cleaner, treatment of ulcer, destroyer of waste flesh
				-Oil	- Treatment of different types of wounds and ulcer
			-Bark	- Infusion	- Treatment of ulcer
	Melia azedarach	Āzād darakht	Leaf, Fruit	Plaster	- Filthy ulcer cleaner
Moraceae	*Morus nigra*	Tut	-Fruit, Leaf -Extract of fruit	-Plaster - Liniment	- Treatment of filthy ulcer - Treatment of ulcer
	Ficus benghalensis	Bara, Lul	Leaf	Plaster	- Warmed leaf: wound healing
	Ficus carica L.	Tin	-Fruit - Leaf	- Plaster - Plaster	-Burnt: blood stopper and ulcer cleaner - Wound healing
	Ficus sycomorus	Jammiz, Shalka anjir	-Sap of Fruit	- Plaster	- Treatment of intractable wound and wound healing
			-Wood	- Powder	-Ash: Treatment of ulcer
	Ficus benghalensis	Raqah yamāni, raqā'	Leaf	Plaster	- Wound healing
Moringaceae	*Moringa aptera Gae.*	Bān, habbo al-bān	Oil of seed	Liniment	- Scar softening
Musaceae	*Musa sp.*	Mawz	Bark, Fruit peel	Powder	- Blood stopper, treatment and ulcer dryer
	Balaustion pulcherrimum	Jolnar, Golnar	Flower	-Powder, Plaster	- Treatment of ulcer - Treatment of wound caused by contusion and cut
Myrtaceae	*Myrtus communis L.*	Ās	Leaf, Fruit	Oral, Plaster, Epithem	- Oil of leaf or fruit: treatment of ulcer - Edema reducer, blood stopper

Family	Scientific name	Traditional name	Part used	Application	Therapeutic effect
Nymphaeaceae	*Nymphaea lotus*	Nilofar	Root, Seed	Plaster	- Treatment of ulcer
	Fraxinus griffithii	Buqisa, Darvan, Dardar	Leaf, Bark, Bloom	-Powder - Plaster	- Astringent, wound healing and treatment of filthy ulcer -Fresh leaf: Treatment of fresh wound
Oleaceae	*Olea europia*	Zeitoon	-Oil of raw olive - Dreg of olive oil -Gum	-Liniment - Plaster - Plaster	- Wound healing and treatment of wet and dry ulcer - Treatment of dry ulcer -Flesh grower and moist wound dryer
	Fraxinus excelsior L.	Lesan ol-asafir	Leaf	Plaster	- Treatment and wet ulcer cleaner and wound healing -Flesh grower
Orchidaceae	*Orchis militaris*	Khusy al-kalb	Root	Plaster, Powder	- Ulcer cleaner - Treatment of filthy ulcer
	Serapias lingua L.	Lanjitos	Root	Plaster	- Wound cleaner and treatment of wound
Pandanaceae	*Pandanus odoratissimus* L.	Kāzi	Wood	Powder	-Wound healing
	Papaver rhoeas L.	Shaqaieq	-Leaf, Stem -Flower	-Liniment -Powder	- Pus cleaner - Pus cleaner ,wound healing and treatment of filthy ulcer
Papaveraceae	*Glaucium flavum*	Khashkhash bahri	Leaf, Flower	-Plaster -Liniment	- Treatment of filthy ulcer, destroyer of waste and rotten flesh -Flower: scar removal
	Papaver somniferum	Khashkhāsh bostāni	Leaf, Flower	-Plaster -Liniment	- Destroyer of intractable ulcer - Flower: scar removal
Papilionaceae	*Astragalus fasciculifolius* Boiss.	Anzarut	Gum	Topical	- Wound healing

Table 1. (Continued)

Family	Scientific name	Traditional name	Part used	Application	Therapeutic effect
Parmeliaceae	*Usnea barbata*	Oshna	Whole plant	Powder	- Flesh grower
	Pinus pinea	Sanobar, Orz	Leaf, Bark	-Decoction -Powder - Liniment -Plaster	-Leaf and bark: Blood stopper - Leaf and bark: wound healing - Leaf and bark: treatment of ulcer and flesh grower - Blood stopper
Pinacea	*Cedrus liibani*	Shorbin	-Resin (Ratinaj, Qatran, Zeft) -Branch -Leaf, Bark - Leaf, bark of root	-Plaster - Decoction -Powder -Oral -Plaster - Liniment	-Strengthening the loose flesh, flesh grower and wound healing -Treatment of ulcer -Blood stopper and Treatment of ulcer - Blood stopper in fresh wound -Fresh leaf: Blood stopper in fresh wound - Treatment of ulcer and intractable ulcer
Piperaceae	*Piper cubeba* L.	Kabāba	Fruit	Plaster	- Treatment of filthy ulcer in soft tissue - Edema reducer - Destroyer of wound and ulcer
	Piper betle L.	Tanbul	Leaf	Plaster	- Blood stopper and wound healing
Plantaginaceae	*Plantago major* L.	Lesān ol-hamal	Leaf, Seed	Powder, Plaster	- Treatment of filthy ulcer and deep wound -Pus cleaner - Siccative and treatment of cancerous and chronic ulcer and deep wound

Family	Scientific name	Traditional name	Part used	Application	Therapeutic effect
Platanaceae	*Platanus orientalis*	Dolb	Leaf	Powder	- Ash: treatment of filthy and peeling skin around the wound - wound and ulcer dryer
	Triticum aestivum	Hentah	Starch	Plaster	- Treatment and healing of ulcer
	Cynodon dactylon	Najm, friz	Leaf	Plaster	- Healing of bloody wound
	Lolium temulentum L.	Shailam	Seed	Plaster, Powder	- Treatment of wound and ulcer
	Oryza sativa L.	Oroz	Seed	Oral	- Ulcer wound -Flesh grower
Poaceae	*Agropyron repens* L.	Thil	-Root, Arial part	-Plaster	- Treatment of fresh and filthy wound -Ash of aerial part: ulcer dryer
	Saccharum officinarum	Sokkar	Extract (sugar)	- Powder	-Blood stopper - Destroyer of waste and rotten flesh and flesh grower
	Arundo arenaria	Qasab	Stem	-Liniment -Plaster	- Treatment of ulcer -Burnt: Treatment of filthy wound
	Polygonum bistorta	Bartāniqi, Sarvāly	Leaf, Extract	Topical	- Wound and ulcer healing
Polygonaceae	*Polygonum equisetiforme*	Asi al-rāei	-Leaf - Extract	-Plaster -Dropping	- Treatment of ulcer and fresh wound - Ulcer dryer
	Rheum rib es	Ribās	Flower	Plaster	Treatment of wound
	Rumex aquaticus L.	Hommāz al-māee, Homāz al-baqar	Arial part	Plaster	- Treatment of wound and cancerous ulcer
Portulocaceae	*Potulaca oleracea*	Baqala hamqā, Khorfeh	Leaf, Stem	Topical	- Treatment of ulcer
Potamogetonaceae	*Potamogeton nataus*	Jār al-nahr	Leaf	Plaster	- Treatment of wet and dry ulcer - Treatment of filthy ulcer

Table 1. (Continued)

Family	Scientific name	Traditional name	Part used	Application	Therapeutic effect
Primulaceae	*Anagallis caerulea Schreb Anagallis arvensis* L.	Ānāghālis	Leaf, Fruit	Plaster	- Wound healing, prevents of wound edema and prevents the spread of ulcer - Thorn and arrow absorber from the body depth
	Cyclamen europaeum	Faqlāminos	Root	Plaster	- Treatment of wound before it gets old - Destroyer of wound
	Lysimachia vulgaris	Lusimākhius	Leaf	Plaster	- Wound healing
Pteridaceae	*Adiantum capillus - veneris* L.	Barshiāoshān, Parsiāvoshān	Leaf	Topical	- Treatment of filthy and wet wound
Punicaceae	*Punica granatum* L.	Rummān	-Seed	-Plaster	- Treatment of filthy ulcer and destroyer of waste flesh
			- Sepal, Peel	-Powder	-Ash or dried: wound dryer and wound healing
			- Boiled and concentrated juice of sour and sweet fruit	-Liniment	- Treatment of chronic and intractable ulcer
Ranunculaceae	*Nigella sativa*	Shuniz	Seed	Plaster	- Treatment of ulcer
	Helleborus niger	Kharbaq aswad	-Sap	-Plaster	- Treatment of fistula and destroyer of rigid wound
			-Root	-Plaster	- Destroyer of waste and rotten flesh
	Delphinium semibarbatum Bi.	Zarir	Flower	Powder	-Ash: wound healing
	Ranunculus sceleratus	Kaffā al-zabo'a	Arial part	Powder	- Destroyer of waste flesh and flesh grower - Wound cleaner and treatment of ulcer

Family	Scientific name	Traditional name	Part used	Application	Therapeutic effect
Rhamnaceae	Zizyphus Spina - Christi	Sedr	Wood filings	Powder	- Treatment of wound
	Ziziphus jujuba	Onnāb	-Leaf -Bark	-Powder -Powder	- Cancerous ulcer remover -Purification and treatment of cancerous wound
	Prunus subg. Prunus	Ijiās	Gum	plaster	- Healing of ulcer
	Cydonia oblonga	Safarjal	-Leaf, Villi of fruit - Fruit	-Plaster, Powder -Oil	- Wound dryer and blood stopper - Treatment of filthy ulcer
	Rasa damascena	Vard	-Bud -Oil	-Powder -Plaster -Liniment	-Dry bud: Thorn and arrow absorber from the body depth and treatment of deep ulcer -Fresh ulcer: flesh grower in deep wound - Wound and ulcer dryer, flesh grower in deep wound
Rosaceae	Pinus comunis	Kummathrā Kummathrā barri (desert pear) Kummathrā hāmez (sour pear)	-Leaf, Wood -Fruit -Fruit	-Powder -Powder -Plaster	-Dry leaf: siccative, healing the wound - Burnt wood and leaf: ulcer dryer - Siccative and wound healing, flesh grower - Unripe fruit: wound healing
	Rubus fruticosus Rubus ulmifolius	Ollaiq	- Fruit, Flower -Fresh leaf, branch	-Liniment -Plaster	- Extract of fresh fruit and flower: prevents the pus flow siccative of wet ulcer, - Treatment of scratch on thigh
	Rosa canina L.	Ollaiq al-kalb	A thing like wool inside the fruit	Plaster	- Wound healing

Table 1. (Continued)

Family	Scientific name	Traditional name	Part used	Application	Therapeutic effect
	Pyrus malus	Tuffāh	Leaf, Fruit, Bark	Plaster	- Astringent - Treatment of ulcer
	Potentilla reptans L.	Khamsa auraq, Bentāfalon	-Leaf	-Plaster -Powder	-Wound healing and blood stopper - Treatment of fresh wound
Rosaceae			-Root	-Decoction	- Treatment of ulcer
	Agrimonia eupatoria	Ghāfeth	Aial part	-Plaster - Powder	- Treatment of intractable ulcer - Siccative and treatment of wound
	Amygdalus amara	Lauz al-mor	-Fruit -Oil	-Plaster -Liniment	- Treatment of old wound - Treatment of wet ulcer
Rubiaceae	*Galium cruciate*	Gāiion	Flower	Plaster	- Blood stopper
Rutaceae	*Ruta graveolens*	Sodāb, Fijen	Leaf	Plaster	- Treatment of old ulcer
Salicaceae	*Populus nigra var. italica*	Gharb	-Leaf, Bark - Flower	- Plaster - Powder	-Fresh leaf and bark: treatment of wet wound -Dry bark: treatment of wound - Siccative of chronic ulcer
Santalaceae	*Viscum album*	Debq	-Berries - Leaf	-Juice - Plaster, Powder	- Treatment of old and filthy ulcer - Treatment of fresh wound
Scrophulariaceae	*Verbascum thapsus*	Busir, Gholumos, Gol-e-māhur	Leaf, Flower	Plaster	- Treatment of wound and ulcer
	Physalis alkekengi L.	Kākanj, Kākna	Shell of fruit, seed	Extract	- Treatment of ulcer
Solanaceae	*Mandragora officinarum*	Serāj al-qotrub	-Seed -Seed, Root	-Plaster - Powder	- Treatment of wound - Treatment of cancerous ulcer

Family	Scientific name	Traditional name	Part used	Application	Therapeutic effect
Solanaceae	Nicotiana tabacum L.	Tanbāku	Leaf	Plaster	-Blood stopper of fresh wound - Siccative of chronic ulcer
	Solanum dulcamara	inab al-tha'lab	Fruit	Plaster	- Prevents the spread of ulcer
Styracaceae	Styrax benzoin	Zerv, Zarv	Wood	Powder	- Blood stopper
Symplocaceae	Symplocos racemosa Roxb	Armak, Armāl	Bark	Topical	- Ulcer dryer -Pus cleaner
Tamaricaceae	Tamarix gallica	Tarfā, Gāz	-Leaf, Branch	-Powder, Ash, Fume	- Siccative of wet ulcer
			-Fruit	-Powder, Ash	-Siccative of filthy ulcer, destroyer of rotten flesh and blood stopper
			-Wood	-Powder	-Ash: treatment of wet ulcer
Thymelaeaceae	Daphne oleoides Daphne mezereum	Māzariun	Leaf	Plaster	- Treatment and cleaner of filthy ulcer
	Daphne gnidium L.	Mathnān	Leaf, Seed	Plaster	- Destroyer of rotten flesh - Treatment and cleaner of filthy ulcer
Urticaceae	Parietaria officinalis	Āzān-ol-far	Whole plant	Plaster	- Wound healing -Wound cleaner - Thorn and arrow absorber from the body depth - Prevents the spread of ulcer and edema
	Urtica urens L.	Anjurah	Leaf, Seed	-Plaster	-Treatment of filthy ulcer and dog bite wound -Ash of leaf: treatment of filthy ulcer
				-Powder	- Siccative of wound
Valerianaceae	Nardostachys jatamansi D.C	Nārdin	Root	Oral	-Wound edema reducer
Verbenaceae	Verbena officinalis L.	Ra'y al-hamām	Leaf	Plaster	- Wound healing - Prevents the spread of ulcer - Treatment of fresh wound - Treatment of deep ulcer

Table 1. (Continued)

Family	Scientific name	Traditional name	Part used	Application	Therapeutic effect
Violaceae	*Viola odorata* L.	Banafsaj	Flower	Oil	- Wound healing
Vitaceae	*Vitis vinifera* L.	Karm	-Branch - Bloom -Fruit	- Plaster - Plaster - Plaster	- Destroyer of waste flesh - Cancerous ulcer remover -Prevents wound edema
Zingiberaceae	*Curcuma Zerumbet*	Jadvār	Root	Powder	-Blood stopper - Wound healing
	Curcuma longa	Oruq sofr	Root	- Plaster, Powder	-Siccative of wound
	Zingiber officinale	Zanjabil	Root	Plaster	-Siccative of old wound
	Tribulus terrestris L.	Hasak	Fruit	Plaster	- Treatment of filthy ulcer - Wound healing
Zygophyllaceae	*Zygophyllum fabago* L.	Amdoriān	Leaf	Powder	- Treatment of fresh wound
	Guaiacum officinale	Gāiac	Wood	Oral (infusion)	- Treatment of cancerous ulcer
Unknown	Unknown	Akharsāj	Leaf, Fruit	Liniment	-Burnt: wound healing
Unknown	Unknown	Bisem	Leaf	Plaster	-Very useful for wound healing
Unknown	Unknown	Buyānas	Root, Gum, Extract	Topical	- Pus cleaner - Removal of rotten bone
Unknown	Unknown	Idmāmir, Idmāmid	Whole plant	Powder	- Blood stopper in old wound -Burnt: blood stopper in old wound and treatment of ulcer

Family	Scientific name	Traditional name	Part used	Application	Therapeutic effect
Unknown	Unknown	Kaliān kātah	Leaf	Topical	- Put the upper surface on the wound: wound healing -Put the lower surface on the wound: destroyer of rotten flesh
Unknown	Unknown	Kasul	Fruit	Powder	- Blood stopper
Unknown	Unknown	Lahuloqu gharāqis	Arial part	Plaster	- Treatment of fresh and old wound
Unknown	Unknown	Lithānulos	Root	Plaster	-Dry root: siccative and treatment of wound and ulcer
Unknown	Unknown	Marsatos	Leaf, Branch	Powder	-Wound healing
Unknown	Unknown	Mojnah	Arial part	-Plaster -Extract	- Blood stopper in fresh wound - Eliminate of wormy ulcer and reduce wound pain
Unknown	Unknown	Shāhsini	Leaf or extract	Powder	- Blood stopper
Unknown	Unknown	Zafar al-qat	Leaf	Plaster	- Wound healing - Treatment of fresh wound
Unknown	Unknown	Zahre	Arial part	Topical	- Treatment of filthy ulcer -Wound healing
Unknown	Unknown	Zajāj	Gum	Plaster	- Destroyer of waste flesh

Table 2. The minerals and natural materials using in TIM for wound healing [5, 12-14]

Traditional name	Common name	Nature	Therapeutic effect
Ābār, Ānk, Rasās aswad	Galena - Primary Lead Ore	Metal	-Treatment of filthy and bad ulcer - Blood stopper - Wound healing
Ājur	Brick	Building material	- Blood stopper
Asābea' ferown	-	Stone	-Blood stopper -Wound healing
Āsyus	Asian stone	Kind of salt on stone near the sea	- Destroyer of rotten flesh -Treatment of deep and large wound
Bāroud	Gunpowder	A mixture of sulfur, charcoal and potassium nitrate	-Blood stopper in fresh wound
Barvāq	-	Stone	-Wound healing
Buraq, Tenkār	Borax	Sodium borate	- Pus cleaner - Destroyer of rotten flesh
Dahanaj	Green malachite	Stone	-Effective for ugly wound
Difurjes	Tutty	Consists of a crude zinc oxide	- Treatment of intractable ulcer
Dik bardik	-	A compound medicine made of lime, orpiment, mercury and verdigris	- Blood stopper - Destroyer of waste flesh, fistula and filthy ulcer
Durdi	Dreg	Lees of wine	- Blood stopper - Wound healing - Destroyer of waste flesh
Ertkān	-	Kind of gravel	- Destroyer of waste flesh - Flesh grower and filling the wound
Esfidāj	Zinc oxide	Powder	- Destroyer of waste flesh - Flesh grower -Siccative of wound

Traditional name	Common name	Nature	Therapeutic effect
Esfidāj al-jassāsin	Gypsum	Calcium sulfate dihydrate	- Blood stopper of fresh wound - Wound healing
Esmed, Kohl, Sorme	Antimony	Stone	- Pus cleaner - Ulcer healing - Destroyer of waste flesh - Blood stopper - Flesh grower
Hajar al-āji, Shekar sang	Marble	Marmar stone like ivory	- Blood stopper
Hajar al-baghar	-	A stone that found in gallbladder of cow	- Wound healing
Hajar al-bohairā	-	A black stone	- Wound healing
Hajar al-esfanj	Sponge stone	A stone that found in sponge	- Blood stopper - Wound healing
Hajar al-habashi, Hajar pelpel	-	A stone like peridot	- Black and green spots remover caused by the wound
Hajar al-labāni	Chalk	Stone	- Blood stopper
Hajar al-loghavā arāfos	-	Stone	- Siccative of wound
Hajar al-meghnātis	Magnet	A stone with magnetism property	- Blood stopper - Wound healing - Treatment of large wound - Very effective in removing poisonous iron tools
Hajar al-namer	-	A stone that forms in leopardess body	- Wound healing
Hajar al-qebti		Stone	- Blood stopper - Wound healing - Prevents the spread of filthy ulcer
Hajar al-qaysur, Hajar al-sha'r	Pierre ponce	A black stone	- Flesh grower
Hajar al-yahud	Jewish stone	laudaikos lithos, lapis judaicus	- Wound healing
Hajar al-zirah	-	Stone	- More effective for wound healing

Table 2. (Continued)

Traditional name	Common name	Nature	Therapeutic effect
Ḥasāt	Calculus	Gravel	- Blood stopper
Kebrīt	Sulphur	Chemical element	- Treatment of wet ulcer
Khabath al- fiddah	Dross	Dross of silver	- Wound healing
Khal	Vinegar	Acetum vinegar	- Prevents the spread of ulcer - prevents of fresh wound edema
Khazaf, Sofāl	Porcelain clay	Clay	- Treatment of ulcer - Wound healing -New sofāl: black and green spots remover caused by the wound
Lāzeward	Lapis lazuli	A deep blue metamorphic rock	- Treatment of ulcer
Lizaq al-dhahab	Chrysocolla	Hydrated copper phyllosilicate mineral	- Treatment of intractable wound
Lu'lu'	Pearl	Composed of calcium carbonate	-Blood stopper and treatment of ulcer
Luqfarlos	Egyptian stone	Stone	- Treatment of ulcer
Maghnisiā	Pyrolusite	Manganese dioxide (MnO2)	- Wound healing
Maisanun	Sea foam	-	-Siccative and treatment of wound and ulcer
Marqashishā	Pyrite, Marcasite	Stone	- Ulcer healing - Destroyer of waste flesh -Flesh grower and treatment of ulcer
Mas haqunia	Dross of glass	The foam that formed in melting process of glass	-Siccative and destroyer of waste rotten flesh of wound
Melh	Salt	Salt (sodium chloride)	- Destroyer of waste flesh - Blood stopper
Melh al-mur	Bitter salt	A compound of magnesium sulfate, sodium sulfate and sodium chloride	-Wound healing

Traditional name	Common name	Nature	Therapeutic effect
Miah al-kebrit	Sulfur water	Water contains a high amount of hydrogen sulfide gas	- Effective for old wound
Mordāsanj	litharge	One of the natural mineral forms of lead(II) oxide, PbO	- Destroyer of waste rotten flesh - Flesh grower - Treatment of deep wound - Ulcer cleaner
Mumia	Mineral pitch	Shilajit	- Treatment of old wound and fistula
Neurah	Quick lime	Calcium oxide	- Destroyer of waste flesh - Wound healing - Blood stopper - Treatment of wound and ulcer - Siccative of wound
Nuhās	Copper	Metal	- Destroyer of waste flesh - Wound healing and healing - Prevents the spread of ulcer - Treatment of hard and cancerous ulcer
Nushādar	Salammoniac	Ammonium chloride	- Blood stopper and siccative of ulcer and wound - Pus cleaner
Nushārah	Wood chips	Small fragments of wood	- Corroded wood chips: wound cleaner and healing - Burnt wood chips: treatment of cancerous and corrosive ulcers and prevents of their infection
Qafr al-yahud	Bitumen judaicum	Asphalt	- Wound edema reducer and prevents wound edema - Wound healing and wound healing - Flesh grower and Eliminates wormy wounds
Qalimia al-dhahab	Litharge of gold	-	- Destroyer of waste flesh - Healing of filthy ulcer - Dirt cleaner and flesh grower of ulcer

Table 2. (Continued)

Traditional name	Common name	Nature	Therapeutic effect
Qalimia al-fiddah	Litharge of silver	-	- Treatment of difficult ulcers - Destroyer of waste flesh - Healing of filthy ulcer - Dirt cleaner and flesh grower of ulcer
Qalqatār, Zāj asfar	Yellow vitriol	Ferric oxide	- Treatment of filthy ulcer - Destroyer of waste flesh
Remād	Ash	Water ash of fig wood	- Treatment of filthy ulcer - Treatment of large and deep ulcer - Destroyer of rotten flesh and flesh grower - Wound healing
Rusokhtaj	-	Burnt copper	- Wound cleaner and healing - Prevents the spread of intractable ulcer - Destroyer of waste and rotten flesh
Shab, Shab yamani	Alum	Hydrated double sulfate salt of aluminium	- Treatment of filthy ulcer - Destroyer of waste flesh - Siccative and Blood stopper
Shādanaj, Hajar hindi	Haematite	Iron oxide	- Destroyer of waste flesh - Treatment of ulcer -Flesh grower - Scar removal - Blood stopper - Treatment of chronic wound and ulcer
Sharab, Mey	Wine	Wine	- Effective for filthy and corrosive ulcer
Tin al-ard al-mazruah	Earth of cultivated land	Clay	- Fresh wound healing -Flesh grower in the ulcer

Traditional name	Common name	Nature	Therapeutic effect
Tin al-maghrah	Red ochre	Clay	- Wound healing
Tin armani	Bole armenian	Clay	- A good wound healing effect
Tin balad mastaki, Tin rumi	Chian earth	Clay	-Wound washing flesh grower
Tin makhtum	Sealing clay	Clay	-Wet ulcer healing - Treatment of difficult ulcers - Treatment of fresh, old and cancerous wound
Tin qaimulia, Andalusia clay, Hajar al-rakhām	Terra cimolia	Clay	- Wound soothing and healing - Treatment of intractable ulcer - Blood stopper -Burnt: treatment of intractable ulcer
Tin qobrosi	Terra cyprica	A red clay from cyprus	-Siccative of ugly wound
Tubal al-nuhās	-	Dross of copper	- Destroyer of waste flesh of wound and Prevents the spread of ulcer
Turāb al-morabbaāt	Intersection's Soil	Soil	-Sicctive and pus cleaner of wound - Wound healing
Tutia	Blue vitriol	Copper sulphate	- Treatment of wound and ulcer - Blood stopper
Zahra al-nuhās	Red oxid of copper	Inorganic compound	- Destroyer of waste flesh of wound - Sicative of wound and filthy ulcer
Zāj akhdar	Green vitriol	Iron(II) sulfate	-Blood stopper
Zanjafr	Cinnabar	Mercuric sulfide	- Treatment of ulcer - Wound healing - Blood stopper -Siccative of wet wound - Flesh grower - Fume: Treatment and siccative of intractable ulcer

Table 2. (Continued)

Traditional name	Common name	Nature	Therapeutic effect
Zanjār, Zangār	Verdigris	Basic acetate of copper	- Wound healing - Prevents the spread of intractable ulcer - Prevents of wound edema -Flesh grower -Cooked with honey: pus cleaner -Burnt: Treatment of all wound on body surface - Destroyer of waste flesh - Correction of filthy intractable ulcer
Zarnikh	Orpiment	Arsenic sulfide	- Destroyer of waste flesh of wound - It is unique in the treatment of different types of wounds
Zeft	Pitch	Derived from petroleum or coal tar	- Ulcer healing - Filthy ulcer cleaner -Siccative of wound
Zibaq	Mercury	Liquid metal	- Treatment of filthy ulcer -Liniment and fume: treatment of intractable wound and ulcer

Table 3. The Animal products using in TIM for wound healing [5, 12-14]

Traditional name	Common name	Nature	Therapeutic effect
Akarea'	Trotter	Trotter of sheep or one year old goat	-Burnt bone: blood stopper
Aqrab	Scorpio	Scorpio	- Burnt: treatment of cancerous and intractable ulcer
Asal al-nahl, shahd	Honey	Honey	-Pus cleaner - Destroyer of waste flesh - Wound healing - Treatment of deep ulcer -Concentrated honey: Treatment of fresh wound
Azfar al-tib	Unguis odoratus	It is a fragrant material consisting of the opercula of certain marine snails	- Treatment of wet wound
Baiz	Egg	Albumen of each bird's egg	- Prevents wound infection
Bār	Dung	-Dung of kamel -Dung of sheep	- Dissolvent of ulcer and favus ulcer - Wound healing
Baul	Urine	-Urine of donkey	- Treatment of wet ulcer
		- Urine of human	- Treatment of wet and deep ulcer, pus cleaner from wound and ulcer, blood stopper
		-Each urine	- If it boiled and concentrated: it is unique in desiccating and healing of cancerous ulcer and fistula
Bolghār	Leather	An aromatic and red leather	- Burnt: Blood stopper of fresh wound
Bussad, Marjān	Coral	Animal	- Destroyer of waste flesh
Buzāq	Saliva	Fasting saliva of human	- Blood stopper and wound healing - Scar removal
Dam	Blood	-Blood of cow - Blood of donkey	- Blood stopper

Table 3. (Continued)

Traditional name	Common name	Nature	Therapeutic effect
Dolā'	Porcupine	Burnt skin	-More effective for wound healing - Treatment of filthy ulcer -Siccative of wound and ulcer - Destroyer of waste flesh
Dud al-harir	Silkworm	Ash of its burnt	-Siccative of wet wound -Wound healing
Esfang	Sponge	Animal	-Treatment of old wound and deep ulcer -Scar removal - Blood stopper
			-Siccative of deep and old wound and ulcer -Burnt esfang: acts stronger in fresh wound healing and stop bleeding
Faras bahri	Hippopotamus	Ash of it	- Siccative of wound -Skin grower
Gharā	Taurocolla	Gelatin, Glue	- Wound edema reducer - Wound healing - Blood stopper
Ghara al-julud	Skin glue	Made from repeated boiling of animal skin	- Wound edema reducer - Blood stopper - Wound healing
Gharā al-samak	Ichtyocolle	Isinglass	-Wound healing

Traditional name	Common name	Nature	Therapeutic effect
Halazun	Snail	Snail slime	- It is unique in treatment of intractable ulcer
Jeld	Skin	-Skin of mule	- Treatment of ulcer without causing edema
		- Skin of sheep	- Fresh skin: treatment of filthy ulcer - Skin chips: blood stopper of fresh wound
		- Oil of rhino skin	- More effective in treatment of wound and ulcer
Jegar, Kabed	Liver	-Ash of donkey liver	- Treatment of ulcer
Jobn	Cheese	-fresh cheese	-Treatment of fresh wound and prevents edema
		-old cheese	- Treatment of bad ulcer
Jund bidastar	Castoreum	Testis of beaver	- Treatment of fatal ulcer
Khaz	Fur	A thick growth of hair that covers the skin of many animals	-Burnt: blood stopper and siccative of wound
Laban	Milk	Milk of cow and goat	- Filthy wound cleaner
Māez	Goat	Animal	- Adipose tissue: flesh grower - Burnt dung: treatment of ulcer
Merārah	Bile	-Bile of cow	-Wound healing
		-Bile of male goat	- Destroyer of waste flesh - Treatment of large old ulcer
		-Bile of black cat	- Treatment of old ulcer
Mum	Beeswax	Natural wax produced by honey bees	- Ulcer cleaner from filth and pus - Wound healing
Namer	Leopard	Meat and Adipose tissue	-Cooked: wound destroyer
Nasj al-ankabut	-Spider's web -Egg sac	Proteinaceous spider silk	- Prevents wound edema - Blood stopper - Wound healing -Siccative of fresh wound and act like suture
Qermez	Cochineal	It is crimson-dye-producing insect	-Wound healing -Treatment of large wound

Table 3. (Continued)

Traditional name	Common name	Nature	Therapeutic effect
Rakhāmah, Nasr	Vulture	-Shell of egg and skin -feather	-Powder: blood stopper and wound healing -Ash of feather: treatment of ulcer
Rish-e-bāzi Rish-e-andalib	Feather	-Feather of falcon - Feather of nightingale	-Burnt: wound healing
Sadaf	Oyster	-Burnt shell - Oyster meat and shell - Oyster meat	- Pus cleaner and treatment of ulcer - Wound healing - Thorn and arrow absorber from the body depth
Samak	Fish	Burnt of dried fish head	- Destroyer of waste flesh of ulcer and prevents the spread of ulcer
Sartān bahri	Sea crab	Burnt shell	- Siccative of wound and filling ulcer -Blood stopper
Shahm al-baqar	Cow's suet	Adipose tissue around the kidney	- Treatment of wound and ulcer
Shahm al-hamām	Pigeon's suet	Adipose tissue around the kidney	- Scar removal
Shahm al-hemār	Ass's suet	Adipose tissue around the kidney	- Scar removal
Sha'r	Hair	-Burnt hair of human - Thin hair of kamel - Burnt hair of Squirrel	- Very effective in drying of wound, cancerous and filthy ulcer, blood stopper -Powder: treatment and ulcer cleaner -Burnt: blood stopper -Powder: blood stopper and wound healing
Suf	Wool	Wool of sheep	- Burnt: Destroyer of waste flesh and treatment of ulcer -Flesh grower -Siccative of wound

Traditional name	Common name	Nature	Therapeutic effect
Sulahfāt	Turtle	Plaster of bone	-Wound healing - Prevents ulcer formation
Tāvous	Peacock	-Blood - Bile	- Treatment of intractable ulcer - Treatment of ulcer and scar removal -Burnt: wound healing
Tehāl	Spleen	Spleen of each animal	-Dried blood of it: blood stopper and wound healing
Vashaq	Lynx	Hair	- Burnt: Treatment of chronic wound
Zabād	Civet	Its musk	- Treatment of ulcer
Zebl	-Dung -Feces	-Dog dung (that has eaten bone) -Dog dung -Cow dung (fresh and warm) - Feces of baby	-Treatment of old ulcer -Dried dung or dung ash: Treatment of old wound -Wound healing, blood stopper and wound edema reducer -If has eaten light food: wound healing
Zebel al-hamām	Pigeon excreta	Pigeon Droppings	- Siccative and treatment of wet wound
Zobd	Butter	Produced from milk of cow, sheep, Goat and Buffalo	- Ulcer cleaner and filler - Wound healing - Flesh grower - Wound and ulcer destroyer if butter washed 101 times with cold water -Putting oil-impregnated cotton on the opening of the wound will spread the opening and purge the wound from the pus

REFERENCES

[1]   Lahlou, Mouhssen. 2004. "Methods to study the phytochemistry and bioactivity of essential oils." *Phytotherapy research* 18(6): 435-48. Accessed July 5, 2019. doi: org/10.1002/ptr.1465.

[2]   Delfan, Bahram, Mahmoud Bahmani, Zohre Eftekhari, Mahyar Jelodari, Kourosh Saki, and Tahereh Mohammad. 2014. "Effective herbs on the wound and skin disorders: a ethnobotanical study in Lorestan province, west of Iran." *Asian Pacific Journal of Tropical Disease* 4: 938-42. Accessed July 5, 2019. doi: org/10.1016/S2222-1808(14)60762-3.

[3]   Ghannadi, Alireza, Behzad Zolfaghari and Shahpour Shamashian. 2011. "Necessity, Importance, and Applications of Traditional Medicine Knowledge in Different Nations." *Journal of Islamic and Iranian Traditional Medicine.* 2(2): 161-76. Accessed July 5, 2019. URL: http://jiitm.ir/article-1-97-fa.html.

[4]   Sedaghat, Reza, Mohammad H. Ghosian Moghadam, Mohsen Naseri, and Ali Davati. 2011. "Histological evaluation of the anti-inflammatory effects of *Alkanna tinctoria* on the cutaneous wounds healing in rat." *Hormozgan Medical Journal* 14 (4):281-89. Accessed July 5, 2019. URL: http://eprints.hums.ac.ir/id/eprint/639.

[5]   Avicenna. 1983. *Al-Qanun fi al-Tibb (The canon of medicine).* Translated by Abdurrahman sharafkandi. Tehran, Iran: Soroush. [In Persian].

[6]   Naseri, Mohsen, Hossein Rezaee Zade, Rasoul Choopani and Magid Anoshiravani. 2012. *An Overview of Traditional Persian Medicine.* Tehran: Traditional Persian Medicine.

[7]   Rameshk, Maryam, Fariba Sharififar, Mitra Mehrabani, Abbas Pardakhty, Alireza Farsinejad and Mehrnaz Mehrabani. 2018. "Proliferation and *In Vitro* Wound Healing Effects of the Microniosomes Containing *Narcissus tazetta* L. Bulb Extract on Primary Human Fibroblasts (HDFs)." *DARU Journal of Pharmaceutical Sciences* 26(1): 31-42. Accessed July 7, 2019. doi: org/10.1007/s40199-018-0211-7.

[8] Ashkani-Esfahani, Soheil, Mohammad H. Imanieh, Mahsima Khoshneviszadeh, Aidin Meshksar, Ali Noorafshan, Bita Geramizadeh, Sedigheh Ebrahimi, Farhad Handjani and Nader Tanideh. 2012. "The healing effect of arnebia euchroma in second degree burn wounds in rat as an animal model." *Iranian Red Crescent Medical Journal* 14(2): 70-4. Accessed July 7, 2019.URL:https://www.ncbi.nlm.nih.gov/pmc/articles/PMC3372044.

[9] Faramarzi, Hossain, Pezhman Bagheri, Ali A. Mohammadi and Effat Hadizadeh. 2012. "Epidemiology of Burn in Fars Province in 2009." *Iranian Journal of Epidemiology* 8(2): 54-64.Accessed July 7, 2019. URL: http://irje.tums.ac.ir/article-1-9-en.html.

[10] Pattanaik, Sovan, Sudam Chandra Si, Abhisek Pal, Jasmin Panda and Siva Shankar Nayak. 2014. "Wound healing activity of methanolic extract of the leaves of Crataeva magna and Euphorbia nerifolia in rats." *Journal of Applied Pharmaceutical Science* 4 (3):46-9. Accessed July 7, 2019. doi: 10.7324/JAPS.2014.40310.

[11] Ghasemi Pirbalouti, Abdollah, Shahrzad Azizi and Abed Koohpayeh. 2012. "Healing potential of Iranian traditional medicinal plants on burn wounds in alloxan-induced diabetic rats." *Revista Brasileira de Farmacognosia* 22(2):397-403. Accessed July 7, 2019. doi:org/10.1590/S0102-695X2011005000183.

[12] Jorjani, Esmail. 2012. *Zakhire Kharazmshahi*. Qom: Institute for Natural Medicine recovery.

[13] Heravi, Movafagh Ibn Ali. 1967. *Alabniyeh - an Haqhiqhe al-Adwiya*. Edited by Ahmad Bahmanyar. Tehran: University of Tehran Press.

[14] Aghili Khorasani, Mohammad Hossein. 2009. *Makhzan al Adviyeh*. Edited by Mohammad Reza Shams Ardakani, Roja Rahimi and Fateme Farjadmand. Tehran: Sabz-arang and Tehran University of Medical Sciences.

Chapter 2

THE ROLE OF ANTIBIOTIC ALTERNATIVES IN CONTROLLING MULTI-DRUG RESISTANT WOUND INFECTIONS

Meera Surendran Nair[1] and Kumar Venkitanarayanan[2],

[1]Department of Veterinary Population Medicine, University of
Minnesota, Saint Paul, MN, US
[2]Department of Animal Science, University of Connecticut,
Storrs, CT, US

ABSTRACT

An injury to skin initiates an array of pathophysiological events,
including inflammation, tissue remodeling, and tissue repair. However,
microbial colonization and invasion of the exposed subcutaneous tissues
with pathogenic microorganisms increase the risk of wound infections.
The threat is even greater when pyogenic wounds are colonized with
antimicrobial resistant pathogens. With almost no new class of antibiotic
drugs in the development pipeline, the use of non-antibiotic antibacterial
agents, including phytochemicals and metals have extensively been

---

* Corresponding Author's E-mail: kumar.venkitanarayanan@uconn.edu.

researched to replace or supplement the current arsenal of antimicrobial medications. Furthermore, the application of phages, the natural bacterial predators, has been found to be effective in resolving chronic multi-drug resistant wound infections. Recently, the primary objective of wound management has been revised to address the role of skin microbiome in acute and chronic wound healing. In light of these new paradigms of microbial ecology and beneficial bacterial interactions, probiotics therapy have also emerged as potential pro-healers aiding tissue repair mechanisms associated with skin abrasions. This chapter will discuss in detail the various antibiotic alternative therapies that could be used against antimicrobial resistant bacteria in wound infections.

INTRODUCTION

Wounds are the reverberations to disruption of normal architecture and function of skin with associated soft tissue layers by trauma or chronic mechanical stress. Essentially, all skin lesions in the clinical care community are called wounds, and they are broadly divided into acute or chronic types. An acute wound could be the result of external trauma or surgical operative procedure and proceeds normally in the healing process. The external manifestations of the healing cascade are often evident in acute wounds without complications. Alternatively, a chronic wound often takes more than three weeks to heal as they fail to produce anatomic and functional integrity in a timely fashion (Bowler, Duerden, & Armstrong, 2001; Bowler, 2009). Wound healing is in fact, a highly regulated process and an injury to the skin initiates an array of pathophysiological events, including inflammation, tissue remodeling, and tissue repair (Gonzalez et al. 2016). Regeneration and tissue repair processes consist of a sequence of molecular and cellular events, which include exudative, proliferative, and extracellular matrix restoration phases. These events occur through the integration of dynamic processes involving soluble mediators, blood cells, and parenchymal cells (Han and Ceilley 2017).

Chronic wounds are a serious public health issue. In the United States, the chronic wounds comprise of 1 to 2 million diabetic foot ulcers, 1 to 2 million venous leg ulcers, 3 to 5 million pressure ulcers, and 1% surgical site infections (Sen et al. 2009; Percival and Cutting 2010). However, comparably acute infections remain less in number. The rapid onset and ability to respond readily and completely to antibiotics define the characterizing clinical feature for acute infections, whereas chronic infections are known to be persistent and recalcitrant (Percival and Cutting 2010). As a result, chronic wound management and prevention of infection represent an area of concern for clinicians and physicians worldwide. Although, both the pathophysiology of wound healing and microbial biofilm development are complex, the combination of the two in chronic wounds makes it a complex biological system, which is dynamic and diverse. On the same line, infection in post-surgical wounds can significantly be influenced by variety of pre-operative and intra-operative procedures. In circumstances where an excessive endogenous bacterial contamination and potential wound infection are expected, broad-spectrum prophylactic antibiotic therapy is recommended (Gottrup 2000; Nichols 2001). Nevertheless, failure to target both aerobic and anaerobic bacteria in acute and chronic mixed infections has been associated with poor clinical outcomes (Gorbach 1994). The risk is even worse when pyogenic wounds are colonized with antimicrobial resistant pathogens.

MICROBIOLOGY OF WOUNDS

Healthy skin is the first line of defense against invading microbes, and it has its own armory to dispose opportunistic microbial penetration (Gallo and Nakatsuji 2011; Grice and Segre 2011). Conversely, skin is one of the largest ecosystems in human body with folds, invaginations and specialized niches that support a wide array of microorganisms (Grice and Segre 2011). The majority of microorganisms found on the skin are called resident flora or indigenous microbiota, which are irreversibly attached to the skin and usually remain dormant, die, or detach after a short period of time (Price 1938; Percival and Cutting 2010). The transient flora is another group of skin microbes generally not found attached to skin and do not persist. They reflect personal hygiene, lifestyle, personal activities and level of environmental contamination (Price 1938; Percival and Cutting 2010). Yet another group is the temporary or nomadic flora. They are able to multiply on the skin surface, but only persist for relatively short periods (Price 1938; Somerville-Millar and Noble 1974). Although gram-positive bacteria are predominately found on the skin surface, gram-negative and fungi population are not rare. Common skin flora includes *Staphylococcus, Micrococcus, Acinteobacter Corynebacterium, Propionibacterium, Malassezia, Dermabacter,* and *Brevibacterium* (Mackowiak 1982; Kong 2011).

The resident flora of normal skin has been found to exist as both planktonic cells and microcolonies on and within the stratum corneum layer, and associated with the sebaceous glands if lipophilic in nature (Somerville and Noble 1973). While both phenotypic states may play an important role in healing and causing infection of acute and chronic wounds, pathogenic biofilms *per se* that are present in all chronic wounds retard healing in a timely fashion (Percival, McCarty, and Lipsky 2015). In a wound bed, the bacteria by default will be surface-associated owing to the availability of nutrient rich surfaces and unavailability of freestanding pools of liquid within which the populations could easily establish a planktonic lifestyle (Percival, McCarty, and Lipsky 2015). Within the biofilm communities, the infectious agents are protected from host defenses and are known to develop resistance to antibiotic treatments. Based on previous studies, biofilms in chronic wounds are mostly polymicrobial and observed to establish quickly in an impaired host, penetrating the surface of the wound (James et al. 2008).

Although hosts and their skin inhabitants do not exhibit mutual dependency, the balance is critical. The commensals display protective function to the skin through various factors such as bacteriocin production, prevention of adherence of competing bacteria, and degradation of pathogenic bacteria (Kong 2011). Conversely, depending upon the multiple determinants of host immunocompetency and microbial virulence, a state of infection could develop when cutaneous wounds are colonized. Therefore, the knowledge of the wound microbiology is always critical as the majority of wound beds are colonized with mixed-organisms, and more importantly the mere presence of a recognized potential pathogen does not necessarily indicate infection. Many microbial and host-related factors are likely to influence wound healing, including bacterial synergy, tissue perfusion or presence of devitalized tissue and all of them needs careful evaluation for successful implementation of wound management tools (Bowler 2009).

CURRENT THERAPEUTIC OPTIONS

Skin breaches irrespective of whether they are accidental (e.g., trauma), or intentional (e.g., surgical) permit the invasion of bacterial pathogens and cause skin and soft tissue infections (SSTIs). In the United States, approximately 14.2 million SSTI-related ambulatory care attendances are reported annually (Hersh 2008). Often, treatment involves administration of a topical antibiotic or antiseptic agent according to specific clinical manifestations. One of the advantages of topical administration is that it offers delivery of high concentrations of antimicrobials at the required site over systemic administration (Williamson, Carter, & Howden, 2017).

Topical antiseptics or biocides have been implicated in the prevention and treatment of localized skin infections over ages. Importantly, they have a broader spectrum of activity and have multiple nonspecific cellular targets. The broader target explains the less propensity of developing resistance in persisting wound associated microbes (Williamson, Carter, and Howden 2017). However, the possible role that these agents may play in driving the emergence of multidrug-resistant pathogens is still unknown. The common antiseptic agents currently in use are povidone-iodine, alcohol, chlorhexidine, triclosan and hydrogen peroxide.

Wound dressings are designed to be in contact with the wound for protecting from contaminations (Dhivya, Padma, and Santhini 2015). Dressing products often include gauze, lint, plasters, bandages and cotton wool (Boateng et al. 2008). Traditionally, such wet-to-dry dressings have been used for wounds requiring debridement. Moisture-retentive dressings

(MRD) have been popular from the 1960s with the understanding that maintenance of a moist wound environment is optimal for healing (Jones, Grey, and Harding 2006). The moist environment has been found to aid granulation tissue formation and regeneration of epithelium, which allow wound fluid containing bactericidal and growth factors to be adjacent to the affected surface to promote debridement (Leaper 1994). However, the risk of increased infections in moist wound conditions prompted clinicians to incorporate antimicrobials in MRDs. Thus, modern wound dressings are being developed not only to facilitate the function of wound healing but also to act as a barrier against penetration of bacteria to the wound environment (Boateng et al. 2008; Dhivya, Padma, and Santhini 2015; Jones, Grey, and Harding 2006).

Antibiotics have been indicated prophylactically for clean, surgical wounds irrespective of the contamination status, whereas for dirty wounds, both prophylactic and therapeutic antibiotic use are indicated (Leaper 1994). Topical antibiotic treatments have been widely used in open wounds; however the emergence of resistant flora following the use of such topical treatments is of concern. Systemic side effects to topical antibiotics are sparse; but allergic reactions on the skin are more frequent. The most common delivery methods for topical application are ointments, cream, lotion, solution, gel, tincture, foam, paste, powder, and impregnated dressings (Heal et al. 2016). Although, several different classes of antibiotics, including mupirocin, bacitracin, neomycin and chloramphenicol are used in clinical practice for topical use, most of them are not intended to systemic application because of known serious adverse effects (Heal et al. 2016). Nevertheless, when the infection is uncontrollable with local interventions, which occurs in extensive cellulitis or deep tissue infections, systemic responses like fever or rigors, osteomyelitis, and sepsis are often observed (Schultz et al. 2003). A few clinical studies have also shown that oral and parenteral therapy for the treatment of SSTIs produced similar clinical and bacteriologic responses (Hernandez 2006). Given the prevalence of antimicrobial resistance, rationalizing the use of antibiotics is critical when selecting empiric therapies for the treatment of an infected chronic wound. Furthermore, the need for the quest of alternatives to antibiotics that have wide spectrum of actions, high margin of safety and a low propensity to induce resistance becomes increasingly important.

The following sections in the chapter will discuss in detail the various antibiotic alternative therapies that could be used against antimicrobial resistant bacteria in wound infections.

PHYTOCHEMICALS IN WOUND HEALING

Medicinal plants have been used as complementary, alternative or integrative therapy for several diseases worldwide. Bioactive products from plants have been used to treat wounds for centuries. The common mechanisms underlying phytochemical-mediated enhanced wound healing include their antioxidant, anti-inflammatory, and antimicrobial effects (Shah and Amini-Nik 2017). In fact, natural antimicrobial agents that act as free-radical neutralizers are found to play an important role in enhancing wound healing (Shah and Amini-Nik 2017).

Curcumin, a polyphenol found in the rhizome of *Curcuma longa* (turmeric), has been investigated widely for the treatment of hyper-inflammatory wounds such as chronic diabetic wounds and burns (Akbik et al. 2014). Additionally, curcumin has potent antioxidant action in cutaneous wounds. Previous studies have demonstrated the suppression of TNF-α and IL-1 production by human macrophages *in vitro* on curcumin administration (Chan 1995). It is also a potent inhibitor of phosphorylase kinase (PhK) and NF-κB activation (Bierhaus et al. 1997; Singh and Aggarwal 1995). Curcumin also has been shown to possess potent antibacterial activity against wound invading pathogens such as *Staphylococcus aureus* and *S. epidermidis* by inhibiting the bacterial FtsZ assembly (Rai et al. 2008). FtsZ is a guanosine triphosphatase that self-assembles into a structure at the bacterial division site termed the "Z ring" (Li et al. 2013). Furthermore, against multidrug-resistant strains of *A. baumannii,* synergistic inhibitory activities were reported with curcumin and epigallocatechin gallate *in vitro* (Betts and Wareham 2014).

Among flavonoids, catechins are one another tested class for their wound healing efficacy (Schmidt et al. 2010). Studies suggested that inhibition of fibroblast growth by flavonoids was found beneficial for the treatment of skin injuries. Luteolin, a flavonoid present in medicinal plants, vegetables and fruits was shown to exert wound healing effects in different wound models (Ozay et al. 2018). Rutin, yet another glycoside flavonoid, was investigated for the ability to enhance production and accumulation of extracellular matrix in healing process (Tran et al. 2011). The antibacterial and astringent activities of flavonoids are known to aid in controlling infections in addition to their antioxidant and anti-inflammatory properties modulating the inflammatory pathways (Antunes-Ricardo, Gutierrez-Uribe, and Serna-Saldivar 2015). Furthermore, the combinatorial activity of an array of flavonoids, including morin, rutin, quercetin, hesperidin, and catechin with antibiotics such as ciprofloxacin, tetracycline, erythromycin, oxacillin, and ampicillin increased the sensitivity of drug-resistant strains of *S. aureus*, including methicillin-resistant *S. aureus* (MRSA) (Abreu et al. 2015).

Honey has been indicated as a topical treatment for chronic wounds and burns for centuries (Majtan 2014). In chronic wounds and burns which are vulnerable to infections, honey has exhibited broad spectrum bacteriostatic and bactericidal activities (Blair et al. 2009; Alam et al. 2014). While eliminating pathogens, honey also maintains a moist environment favorable to wound healing activities. Honey inhibits cyclooxygenase-2 (COX-2), inducible nitric oxide synthase (iNOS), TNF-α and IL-6 expression (Blair et al. 2009; Hussein et al. 2012). It helps to reduce the degradation of extracellular matrix in chronic wounds by exerting its anti-inflammatory effects (Majtan et al. 2013). Furthermore, to counteract the free-radicals found in chronic wounds, honey maintains a high level of flavonoids, phenolic acids, catalase, peroxidase, carotenoids, and ascorbic acid in the environment (Shah and Amini-Nik 2017). In human clinical trials, honey has shown to enhance angiogenesis and fibroblast proliferation (Molan 2001).

Further it was also shown that using a medical-grade honey, eight common wound infection associated bacterial pathogens, including MRSA, *Acinetobacter, Serratia, Klebsiella* and *Pseudomonas* were inactivated (Blair et al. 2009). These findings collectively have supported the use of honey as an effective topical antimicrobial agent against multi-drug resistant wound infections.

Essential oils (EOs) have been validated for their antimicrobial and regenerative properties in several *in vitro* and *in vivo* wound studies. Various constituents such as cinnamaldehyde, geraniol, thymol, menthol, eugenol and carvacrol have been proven to possess antimicrobial and antibiofilm potential in wound infections (Semeniuc, Pop, and Rotar 2017; Karumathil, Surendran-Nair, and Venkitanarayanan 2016). Generally, EOs are shown to attack lipids and phospholipids existing in bacterial cell membranes and cell walls, impairing the ATP biosynthesis, DNA transcription as well as protein synthesis causing the cytoplasm outflow (Negut, Grumezescu, and Grumezescu 2018; Nair and Kollanoor Johny 2017). Additionally, EOs impede the dynamic transport of nutrients through cell membrane, and coagulation of bacteria cell matters (Negut, Grumezescu, and Grumezescu 2018). EOs have also found to possess negligible effect on the development of antimicrobial resistance compared to antibiotics. Several studies have reported the efficacy of thyme, peppermint, lavender, cinnamon, tea tree, rosemary, eucalyptus, and lemongrass in fighting multidrug wound pathogens such as *A. baumannii* (Sienkiewicz et al. 2014). In simulated wound models, in addition to the antibiofilm effect of trans-cinnamaldehyde and carvacrol, a significant decrease in attachment and invasion of multi-drug resistant *A. baumannii* to wound collagen matrix was observed (Karumathil, Surendran-Nair, & Venkitanarayanan, 2016). These EOs also increased the sensitivity of the bacterium to different classes of antibiotics, indicating the potential therapeutic opportunity for antibiotic-adjuvant therapy (Karumathil et al. 2018). The wound dressings impregnated with EOs have been observed to be biocompatible and augmented healing by suppressing wound infections (Liakos et al. 2015).

ANTIMICROBIAL METALS IN WOUND HEALING

Metal-based antimicrobial agents have received much interest with dramatic increase in the prevalence of drug resistance among wound pathogens. In fact, trace essential metals such as zinc, copper and selenium are linked to wound healing. The angiogenic property of copper and its ability to induce vascular endothelial growth factor in wounds have been documented (Sen et al. 2002). Similarly, the zinc-dependent metzincins are known to play a role in enhancing keratinocyte movement over the wound bed (Lansdown et al. 2007). The role of selenium in improving the antioxidant activity of glutathione peroxidase and in the activation of cytoprotective selenoproteins in the cascade of wound healing received research attention (Sengupta et al. 2010). The redox-active transition metals like copper often participate in the Fenton reaction, resulting in the production of reactive oxygen species, causing oxidation and depletion of microbial antioxidant reservoirs (Mohandas et al. 2018). Additionally, silver is known to have a high affinity with electronegative polymeric membranes of bacteria (Lemire, Harrison, and Turner 2013). Silver (Ag) elaborates broad-spectrum antimicrobial activity which has been well demonstrated against a wide-range of pathogens (Kadam et al. 2019). Silver particles have shown to bind cell wall, cell membrane, DNA and enzymes of bacterial cells. Additional antimicrobial mechanisms include the formation of free radicals and interference with respiratory chain enzymes leading to bacterial cell death. Through destabilizing intermolecular adhesion forces, silver has been shown to disrupt extracellular polymeric matrices of bacterial biofilms (Chaw, Manimaran, and Tay 2005).

Multi-drug resistant *Pseudomonas aeruginosa* biofilm is commonly associated with chronic wound infections and cause delay in healing. Silver-zinc redox-coupled electroceutical wound dressing was observed to disrupt the bacterial biofilms. In addition, the wound dressing accelerated keratinocyte migration and facilitated wound closure (Banerjee et al. 2015). As bacterial biofilms are key contributors to wound colonization and infection, medicated antimicrobial dressings demonstrated to prevent biofilm formation are widely used in SSTIs. For instance, in the case of *A. baumannii* and *P. aeruginosa* wound infections; several silver-containing antimicrobial dressings were tested to possess effectiveness in reducing biofilm formation (Halstead et al. 2015). Cavanagh and co-authors reported greater antimicrobial effects with different types of silver impregnated dressings against *S. aureus* and concentrated surfactant gel with 1% silver sulfadiazine exerted antimicrobial as well as antibiofilm efficacy against *A. baumannii in vitro* (Cavanagh, Burrell, and Nadworny 2010). Similarly using *in vitro* disc diffusion and time kill-kinetic assays, seven different silver-containing dressings were evaluated for their antimicrobial efficacy against seventeen pathogenic microorganisms often associated with pyogenic wound infections, including MRSA, vancomycin-resistant *Enterococcus*, multi drug-resistant *P. aeruginosa* and *Acinetobacter* (Gallant-Behm et al., 2005). Although, there is no correlation between log reduction observed in the time-kill assay and zone of inhibition results, for silver in this study, a significant antimicrobial effect was observed with the different dressings against the array of pathogens tested (Gallant-Behm et al., 2005).

Copper (Cu) is an essential trace element known to possess potent biocidal properties. The biocidal activity of copper has been described by its ability to induce alteration of proteins and inhibition of their biological assembly and activity, plasma membrane permeabilization, and membrane lipid peroxidation (Borkow and Gabbay 2005). Copper salts have been shown to be effective against both gram-positive and gram-negative, antibiotic resistant bacteria isolated from wound infections (Febré et al. 2016). Introducing copper salts into wound dressings not only reduced the risk of wound contamination but also released copper directly into the wound site inducing angiogenesis and skin regeneration (Borkow, Gabbay, and Zatcoff 2008; Borkow et al. 2010). Additionally, a copper complex ([Cu(56Me$_2$phen)(*SS*-dach]Cl$_2$) demonstrated enhanced inactivating and inhibiting effects against MRSA biofilms compared to antibiotics such as vancomycin. This study suggested that the nuclease activity of Cu(II) compounds mediated the anti-biofilm activity against MRSA (Beeton, Aldrich-Wright, and Bolhuis 2014). The importance of copper in wound healing was also well demonstrated by its positive effects in cases of severe burn trauma in children and in the management of phosphorus burns (Chou et al. 2001; Cunningham, Leffell, and Harmatz 1993).

Iron (Fe) has been shown to play a critical role in the pathogenesis of *A. baumannii* wound infections. Acinetobactin, is a major siderophore in *A. baumanni* which chelates iron with extremely high affinity from the wound milieu, and the pathogen's virulence activation system relies on its ability to respond to iron limitation in host tissues (Song et al. 2007; Gaddy et al. 2012). Henceforth, wounds washed out with $FeCl_3$ solution following *A. baumannii* inoculation, did not develop infections, as excess of iron promoted the ubiquitination and stabilization of host master transcriptional regulator HIF1α, and shut down the expression of bacterial virulence factors (Fleming et al. 2017).

Gallium (Ga) is a transition metal with similar valence to iron (Fe^{+3}) and allows the competition with Fe^{3+} binding to iron-requiring enzymes, proteins, and microbial siderophores. Therefore, it acts as an inhibitor to bacterial virulence components requiring iron. This property of gallium has been utilized for illustrating its antimicrobial property against *A. baumannii* (García-Quintanilla et al. 2013). Ga $(NO_3)_3$, the active component of an FDA-approved drug (Ganite), was reported to delay the entry of *A. baumannii* into the exponential phase and reduced bacterial growth. In this study, 58 different *A. baumannii* strains were reported to be inactivated *in vitro* using $Ga(NO_3)_3$ at concentrations ranging from 2 to 80 μM (Antunes et al. 2012). Subcutaneous and topical applications of gallium *in vivo*, for the prevention and treatment of wound infections caused by *S. aureus, A. baumannii* and *P. aeruginosa* have been documented (Bonchi et al. 2014). In thermally injured mouse model, subcutaneous application of gallium maltolate was effective in reducing *S. aureus* as well as other frequent colonizers of burn wounds such as *A. baumannii* and *P. aeruginosa* (DeLeon et al. 2009). Biofilm perturbing effects were also observed using $Ga(NO3)_3$ on preformed biofilms of *Burkholderia cepacia* complex species and *P. aeruginosa* (Banin et al. 2008; Bonchi et al. 2014).

Zinc (Zn) is another trace element known to play critical role in wound healing. The deficiency of zinc in the host tissue has been shown to delay the physiological process of wound healing. Meanwhile, topical application of zinc and its salts exerted improved antibacterial responses when exposed to multi-drug resistant wound infections (Heal et al. 2016). Zinc-containing products demonstrated improved re-epithelialization, reduced inflammation and bacterial growth. In addition, topical zinc oxide application has been used as a debridement agent in the management of burns. Compared to bacitracin, neomycin, polymyxin B, nystatin-neomycin, and thiostrepton-triamcinolone, zinc gluconate enhanced wound healing time and produced greater epithelial regeneration effect on surgically created cutaneous wounds in mice (Kaufman et al. 2014). Blanchard and co-authors screened 34 antimicrobials from a FDA-approved drug library to identify the compounds that had a greater propensity to improve clearance of wound associated bacterial pathogens. Among them, zinc pyrithione was shown to reduce the levels of *A. baumannii* and *S. aureus* biofilm-associated bacteria and exhibited an additive effect in combination with silver sulfadiazine in wound site infections (Blanchard et al. 2016). Additionally, zinc salts were reported to inhibit the adhesion and invasion of MRSA to human keratinocyte cells at their sub-inhibitory and minimum inhibitory concentrations (Lau 2017).

A novel organo-selenium coated bandages showed inhibition of biofilm formation on laboratory strains and clinical isolates of *S. aureus*, *P. aeruginosa* and *S. epidermidis* (Tran et al., 2014). Studies have shown that selenium supplementation could enhance immune responses to *S. aureus in vivo*. Selenium acted in a dose-dependent manner on bacterial inactivation, phagocytosis and macrophage activation (Aribi et al. 2015). In one of the recent studies, at sub-inhibitory concentration (antimicrobial concentration which are neither bactericidal nor bacteriostatic), selenium increased *A. baumannii* sensitivity to five different classes of antibiotics along with reducing bacterial adhesion to human keratinocytes. Further selenium inhibited biofilm formation of *A. baumannii* on simulated wound model (Surendran Nair et al. 2016 ASM abstract; Surendran Nair et al. 2019).

NANOPARTICLES BASED WOUND DRESSINGS

The development of 'nanoantimicrobials' to decrease antibiotic dependence and to manage antimicrobial resistance has gained increased significance in wound management. Antimicrobial nanoparticles (NPs) offer an effective strategy owing to the micron-size and large surface area which enhance their ability to enter cells and prolong the biologically activity (Seil and Webster 2012; Yah and Simate 2015).

Silver NPs have been shown to promote various wound healing attributes, including fibroblast migration and macrophage activation (Kadam et al. 2019). Additionally, *in vitro* and *in vivo* effects of silver nanoparticles in inhibiting and inactivating biofilms of wound pathogens hold their great potential for clinical management in chronic wounds (You et al. 2017). In one of the *in vivo* studies, hydrogels loaded with silver NPs coated with polyethylene glycol were evaluated for their efficacy in a MRSA mouse wound infection model. The hydrogels exhibited consistent bacterial load reduction over 15 days, in addition to its enhanced effects on healing and epithelial restoration (Mekkawy et al. 2017). Combinations of silver NPs and antibiotics such as aztreonam also demonstrated synergy in preventing the *P. aeruginosa* biofilm recovery following treatment, with appreciable defects in biofilm architecture.

Zinc oxide-NPs have also exhibited antimicrobial ability against both gram-positive and gram-negative bacterial pathogens such as *E, coli, Salmonella, Listeria monocytogenes* and *S. aureus* (Anju Manuja 2015). Zinc oxide-NPs interact with membrane lipids causing loss of membrane integrity, penetrate into bacterial cells, resulting in the production of toxic oxygen radicals, which damage DNA, cell membranes or cell proteins, and affect the permeability of bacterial membranes resulting in the inhibition of cell growth, and cell death (Applerot et al. 2009; Raghupathi, Koodali, and Manna 2011). Furthermore, selective toxicity of these NPs to bacteria, exhibiting minimal effects on human cells, suggesting their potential as nanomedicine-based wound therapeutics (Reddy et al. 2007). In a mouse wound infection model, as comparable to antibiotics, zinc oxide-NPs were effective in reducing superficial and deep *S. aureus* bacterial load 7 days post-infection (Golbui Daghdari et al. 2017). However, a combination treatment with chitosan, zinc and copper nanoparticles was effective in rapidly eliminating MRSA wound infection as early as 3 days post-infection (Babushkina, Mamontova, and Gladkova 2015).

Copper NPs were found to cause multiple toxic effects such as generation of reactive oxygen species, lipid peroxidation, protein oxidation and DNA degradation in *E. coli* (Chatterjee, Chakraborty, and Basu 2014). Moreover, copper ions have been reported to regulate the activity and expression of proteins involved in the wound repair process (Kornblatt, Nicoletti, and Travaglia 2016). Selenium NPs have also been tested on wound bacterial strains (*S. aureus, Escherichia coli*, MRSA) which were shown to be more valuable matrix for the use of the wound products in practice (Hegerova et al. 2015).

PHAGES IN WOUND HEALING

Pathogenic bacterial invasion, colonization and biofilm formation suppress the healing ability of chronic wounds. The increased persistence of multi-drug resistant bacteria in chronic wound beds urged the need for development of complementary and alternative effective strategies to antibiotics for treatment. The motivation for such alternative approaches led to reevaluation of the efficacy of phage therapy in supporting the wound management.

Bacteriophages are viruses that specifically infect bacteria, injecting their DNA into prey cells, thereby infecting them. The infecting lytic phage multiplies to form new virus particles, get released by lysis and kills the bacterial cells (Alisky et al. 1998). Bacteriophages have recently been extensively studied as therapeutic agents for acute and chronic burn as well as wound infections, alone or in conjunction with other therapeutics (Rose et al. 2014).

Using both *in vivo* models and limited number of clinical trials, phage therapy has demonstrated as a promising approach in control of cutaneous planktonic and biofilm forms of *P. aeruginosa* and *S. aureus*. Following are some of the appreciable advantages for phages compared to antibiotics: 1) high specificity of bacterial strains a particular phage can infect, because its infectivity is greatly dependent on cell surface interactions. This enables phage-mediated elimination of pathogenic bacteria, whilst preserving resident beneficial flora at the site of infection, 2) ability to fight against multi-drug resistant pathogens, 3) greater effectiveness to planktonic and biofilm cells. Phage infections induce the production of enzymes, including phage-encoded depolymerase and alginase from host cells, that break down biofilm matrix elements (Chan and Abedon 2014), 4) low potential for adverse side effects, 5) bacteriophages can infect persister variants of bacteria when the dormant cells switch to growth mode (Bertozzi Silva, Storms, and Sauvageau 2016). However, there are some drawbacks with phages as well, which include narrow host range, bacterial resistance to phage, the potential for phage-encoded virulence genes that can incorporate into the host bacterial genome, impure phage preparations could contain endotoxin and the host immune system could inactivate phages (Donlan 2009). Alternatively, to overcome the obstacles and, to expand the spectra of activity and improve their efficacy, phages are used as a cocktail or in combination with other antimicrobials. Reports on synergistic antibacterial activities while using phages in combination with antibiotics are promising for the development of complementary strategies to antibiotics for the treatment of chronic wounds.

A combination of phage PEV20 and ciprofloxacin against clinical *P. aeruginosa* strains enhanced biofilm eradication and facilitated epithelial regeneration in wound patients. Additionally, administration of phages reported to lower the required antibiotic concentration to treat the infection (Chang et al. 2019). Effectiveness of new isolates of phages collected from a wastewater treatment plant was investigated for its antibiofilm ability against *P. aeruginosa*, *A. baumannii* and *E. coli* isolates from chronic wounds on porcine skin explants. Single phages and mixtures caused significant reductions in the number of biofilm associated viable cells on porcine skins (Milho et al. 2019).

In vivo studies have used multiple dosages and phage cocktails to establish efficacy against preformed biofilms (Kadam et al. 2019; Mendes et al. 2013; Seth et al. 2013). A cocktail of lytic bacteriophages was administered for up to 8 days post-infection in rodent and pig chronic wound models infected with *S. aureus, P. aeruginosa* and *A. baumanii* (Mendes et al. 2013). Results indicated that topically administered bacteriophages decreased pathogen colonization after 4 days of infection, promoting resolution of the chronic infection. Furthermore, it was reported that phage treatment in combination with wound debridement significantly reduced bacterial burden (Seth et al. 2013). As wound debridement occurs in the standard practice of wound care, the combination with phages enables the possibility to improve overall therapeutic outcomes.

Several clinical trials have been pursued recently, evaluating the usage and safety of phages for infected wounds in humans, particularly on burn and post-surgical infections (Furfaro, Payne, and Chang 2018). Interestingly, a recent clinical trial revealed the potential efficacy of topical cocktail bacteriophage therapy for the treatment of chronic wounds with *E. coli, S. aureus*, and *P. aeruginosa*. Patients with chronic nonhealing wounds, not responding to conventional local debridement and antibiotic therapy were enrolled in the study. After administering 3 to 5 doses of bacteriophages topically, significant improvement was observed in the wound healing with no signs of infection. It was found that 35% of enrolled patients achieved complete healing by day 21 while in others, healthy margins and healthy granulation tissue were observed (Gupta et al. 2019). Recently, in another randomized phase trial, the efficacy and tolerability of a cocktail of lytic anti- *P. aeruginosa* bacteriophages (PhagoBurn) compared with standard of care for patients with burns. Although, at the low concentrations tested, the cocktail was reported to reduce bacterial burden in infected wounds, the effect was slower than the standard of care (Jault et al. 2019).

SKIN MICROBIOME IN WOUND HEALING

The physical disruption of tissues begins as an inflammatory response and wound healing is a multi-layered sequential process. The recent advances in the growing field of microbiome analysis have revealed relative amounts of different bacterial flora in different types of wounds (Singer and Clark 1999; Zeeuwen et al. 2013). However, there remains a considerable amount to discover regarding the role of skin dysbiosis in wound healing. Walcott et al. and James et al. demonstrated that *Staphylococcus* and *Pseudomonas* were the common bacterial types in all chronic wound types (Wolcott et al. 2016; James et al. 2008). However, gram-negative rods were reported to be most abundant in the case of biofilm formation. Anaerobic bacteria have also been found to have a regular presence in chronic wounds more than acute wounds. Anaerobes such as *Fingelodia, Prevotella, Peptonipihlus, Peptostreptococcs,* and *Anaerococcus* have been identified as consistent microbial members of the chronic wound microbiome (Wolcott et al. 2016; James et al. 2008). The changes in cutaneous microbiome were also found to associate with acute wounds like burn wounds. It was observed that imbalances in skin microbiome (dysbiosis) as one of the expected consequences of burn injury, which was shown to persist even after healing (Liu et al. 2018). In previous studies, *Corynebacterium* demonstrated a positive correlation with burn wound infection, and *Staphylococcus* and *Propionibacterium* demonstrated a negative correlation with post burn infection (Plichta et al. 2017; Liu et al. 2018).

Altogether, diverse mechanistic insights into the association of the altered microbiome and wounds have paved the way for preclinical studies, including animal models and *in vitro* systems to understand the effects of bacterial colonization on skin inflammation and in developing improved biological interventions. For instance, murine wound models reinforced our understanding on how *Staphylococcus* biofilms delayed wound re-epithelization in uninfected wounds through quorum sensing (Schierle et al. 2009). Taken from here, quorum sensing inhibitors, have shown to be effective in restoring cutaneous integrity of such wounds, abolishing biofilm formation and eliminating bacterial bioburden as well as an attractive adjuvant to antibiotics to combat the development of antibiotic resistance (Kalia 2013; Schierle et al. 2009). An array of studies then supported the consensus that the inhibition of microbial quorum sensing is successful at limiting biofilm formation and improving wound healing (Scutera, Zucca, and Savoia 2014).

Furthermore, with increasing concerns on antibiotic resistance, finding alternative ways to modulate the microbiome to improve wound healing is of the utmost importance. Such clinical applications targeting the microbiome have already been demonstrated in atopic dermatitis (AD) cases. Microbial ecology dynamics showed that AD lesions have a reduced abundance of skin commensals, resulting in decreased production of antimicrobial peptides (Williams and Gallo 2015). Subsequently, treatment with topical application of *Lactobacillus johnsonii* and *Vitreoscilla filiformis* along with reintroduction of antimicrobial peptides improved the healing of skin lesions in AD patients (Nakatsuji et al. 2016; Blanchet-Réthoré et al. 2017; Gueniche et al. 2008). Additionally, short chain fatty acids (SCFAs) produced by skin commensals have demonstrated antimicrobial properties. The administration of SCFAs such as acetic, butyric, and propionic acid suppressed skin inflammation by activating cutaneous T-regulatory cells (Tregs) in a histone acetylation dependent mechanism (Schwarz, Bruhs, and Schwarz 2017).

PROBIOTICS IN WOUND HEALING

There is an increasing interest in using probiotic organisms to restore the skin microbiome and improve cutaneous healing. In *Pseudomonas* colonization and infection, *Lactobacillus plantarum* containing probiotics inhibited the production of elastase, biofilms, and acyl homoserine lactone by the pathogen and improved tissue repair in a burn mouse model (Valdéz et al. 2005). Furthermore, Argenta and co-authors demonstrated that *L. plantarum* administration was able to cause an 80% decrease in mortality in a *Pseudomonas*-infection porcine burn model (Argenta et al. 2016). *S. epidermidis* was found to increase production of poly-ethylene glycol dimethacrylate, an inductor of SCFAs, aiding the decolonization of MRSA strain in infected skin wounds in rodents (Kao et al. 2017). Furthermore, a skin-gut axis was established by supplementing the lactic acid bacterium,

L. reuteri in drinking water, accelerating cutaneous wound healing process in animals. The mechanism was mediated by bacteria-induced oxytocin-activated FoxP3+CD25+host immune Tregs, which decreased the inflammatory damage caused by the innate immune system and led to increased collagen deposition rates (Poutahidis et al. 2013).

CONCLUSION

Control of wound infection today is relied on an array of antibiotic alternatives as mentioned in the chapter, foreseeing the prospect of a post-antibiotic era. A plethora of research supports the development and potential use of such interventions in order to maintain and extend the antimicrobial armamentarium. Majority of the non-conventional therapies are also gaining interest as valuable adjuncts to current standard of care approaches in wound management, for instance, the usage of bacteriophages, and probiotics along with current antibiotics. Recently, antimicrobial metal nanoparticles have gained significant interest particularly in broad-spectrum medicated wound dressing applications. One of the major advantages with the antibiotic alternatives is their mode of action affecting multiple cellular target sites in a non-specific way unlike the antibiotics, which in turn reduces the likelihood of selecting for resistant strains of wound pathogens. Therefore, to explore the possibilities, it would be critical to evaluate these approaches in clinical studies in addition to *in vivo* platforms both alone and in combination with conventional wound management practices.

REFERENCES

Abreu, Ana Cristina, Sofia C. Serra, Anabela Borges, Maria José Saavedra, Andrew J. Mcbain, António J. Salgado, and Manuel Simoes. "Combinatorial activity of flavonoids with antibiotics against drug-resistant *Staphylococcus aureus.*" *Microbial Drug Resistance* 21, no. 6 (2015): 600-609.

Akbik, Dania, Maliheh Ghadiri, Wojciech Chrzanowski, and Ramin Rohanizadeh. "Curcumin as a wound healing agent." *Life sciences* 116, no. 1 (2014): 1-7.

Alam, Fahmida, M. D. Islam, Siew Hua Gan, and Md Khalil. "Honey: a potential therapeutic agent for managing diabetic wounds." *Evidence-Based Complementary and Alternative Medicine* (2014).

Alisky, J., K. Iczkowski, A. Rapoport, and N. Troitsky. "Bacteriophages show promise as antimicrobial agents." *Journal of Infection* 36, no. 1 (1998): 5-15.

Antunes, Luísa CS, Francesco Imperi, Fabrizia Minandri, and Paolo Visca. "*In vitro* and *in vivo* antimicrobial activities of gallium nitrate against multidrug-resistant *Acinetobacter baumannii.*" *Antimicrobial agents and chemotherapy* 56, no. 11 (2012): 5961-5970.

Antunes-Ricardo, Marilena, Janet Gutierrez-Uribe, and Sergio O Serna-Saldivar. "Anti-inflammatory glycosylated flavonoids as therapeutic agents for treatment of diabetes-impaired wounds." *Current topics in medicinal chemistry* 15, no. 23 (2015): 2456-2463.

Applerot, Guy, Anat Lipovsky, Rachel Dror, Nina Perkas, Yeshayahu Nitzan, Rachel Lubart, and Aharon Gedanken. "Enhanced antibacterial activity of nanocrystalline ZnO due to increased ROS-mediated cell injury." *Advanced Functional Materials* 19, no. 6 (2009): 842-852.

Argenta, Anne, Latha Satish, Phillip Gallo, Fang Liu, and Sandeep Kathju. "Local application of probiotic bacteria prophylaxes against sepsis and death resulting from burn wound infection." *PloS one* 11, no. 10 (2016): e0165294.

Aribi, Mourad, Warda Meziane, Salim Habi, Yasser Boulatika, Hélène Marchandin, and Jean-Luc Aymeric. "Macrophage bactericidal activities against *Staphylococcus aureus* are enhanced *in vivo* by selenium supplementation in a dose-dependent manner." *PloS one* 10, no. 9 (2015): e0135515.

Babushkina, I. V., I. A. Mamontova, and E. V. Gladkova. "Metal nanoparticles reduce bacterial contamination of experimental purulent wounds." *Bulletin of experimental biology and medicine* 158, no. 5 (2015): 692-694.

Banerjee, Jaideep, Piya Das Ghatak, Sashwati Roy, Savita Khanna, Craig Hemann, Binbin Deng, Amitava Das, Jay L. Zweier, Daniel Wozniak, and Chandan K. Sen. "Silver-zinc redox-coupled electroceutical wound dressing disrupts bacterial biofilm." *PloS one* 10, no. 3 (2015): e0119531.

Banin, Ehud, Alina Lozinski, Keith M. Brady, Eduard Berenshtein, Phillip W. Butterfield, Maya Moshe, Mordechai Chevion, Everett Peter Greenberg, and Eyal Banin. "The potential of desferrioxamine-gallium as an anti-*Pseudomonas* therapeutic agent." *Proceedings of the National Academy of Sciences* 105, no. 43 (2008): 16761-16766.

Beeton, Michael L., Janice R. Aldrich-Wright, and Albert Bolhuis. "The antimicrobial and antibiofilm activities of copper (II) complexes." *Journal of inorganic biochemistry* 140 (2014): 167-172.

Bertozzi Silva, Juliano, Zachary Storms, and Dominic Sauvageau. "Host receptors for bacteriophage adsorption." *FEMS microbiology letters* 363, no. 4 (2016).

Betts, Jonathan W., and David W. Wareham. "*In vitro* activity of curcumin in combination with epigallocatechin gallate (EGCG) versus multidrug-resistant *Acinetobacter baumannii*." *BMC microbiology* 14, no. 1 (2014): 172.

Bierhaus, Angelika, Youming Zhang, Peter Quehenberger, Thomas Luther, Michael Haase, Martin Müller, Nigel Mackman, Reinhard Ziegler, and Peter P. Nawroth. "The dietary pigment curcumin reduces endothelial tissue factor gene expression by inhibiting binding of AP-1 to the DNA and activation of NF-κB." *Thrombosis and haemostasis* 77, no. 04 (1997): 772-782.

Blair, S. E., N. N. Cokcetin, E. J. Harry, and D. A. Carter. "The unusual antibacterial activity of medical-grade Leptospermum honey: antibacterial spectrum, resistance and transcriptome analysis." *European journal of clinical microbiology & infectious diseases* 28, no. 10 (2009): 1199-1208.

Blanchard, Catlyn, Lauren Brooks, Katherine Ebsworth-Mojica, Louis Didione, Benjamin Wucher, Stephen Dewhurst, Damian Krysan, Paul M. Dunman, and Rachel AF Wozniak. "Zinc pyrithione improves the antibacterial activity of silver sulfadiazine ointment." *mSphere* 1, no. 5 (2016): e00194-16.

Blanchet-Réthoré, Sandrine, Valérie Bourdès, Annick Mercenier, Cyrille H. Haddar, Paul O. Verhoeven, and Philippe Andres. "Effect of a lotion containing the heat-treated probiotic strain *Lactobacillus johnsonii* NCC 533 on *Staphylococcus aureus* colonization in atopic dermatitis." *Clinical, cosmetic and investigational dermatology* 10 (2017): 249.

Boateng, J.S., Matthews, K.H., Stevens, H.N. and Eccleston, G.M., 2008. Wound healing dressings and drug delivery systems: a review. *Journal of pharmaceutical sciences*, 97(8), pp.2892-2923.

Bonchi, Carlo, Francesco Imperi, Fabrizia Minandri, Paolo Visca, and Emanuela Frangipani. "Repurposing of gallium-based drugs for antibacterial therapy." *Biofactors* 40, no. 3 (2014): 303-312.

Borkow, Gadi, and Jeffrey Gabbay. "Copper as a biocidal tool." *Current medicinal chemistry* 12, no. 18 (2005): 2163-2175.

Borkow, Gadi, Jeffrey Gabbay, and Richard C. Zatcoff. "Could chronic wounds not heal due to too low local copper levels?" *Medical hypotheses* 70, no. 3 (2008): 610-613.

Borkow, Gadi, Jeffrey Gabbay, Rima Dardik, Arthur I. Eidelman, Yossi Lavie, Yona Grunfeld, Sergey Ikher, Monica Huszar, Richard C. Zatcoff, and Moshe Marikovsky. "Molecular mechanisms of enhanced wound healing by copper oxide-impregnated dressings." *Wound repair and regeneration* 18, no. 2 (2010): 266-275.

Bowler, P. G., B. I. Duerden, and David G. Armstrong. "Wound microbiology and associated approaches to wound management." *Clinical microbiology reviews* 14, no. 2 (2001): 244-269.

Bowler, Philip G. "Wound pathophysiology, infection and therapeutic options." *Annals of medicine* 34, no. 6 (2002): 419-427.

Cavanagh, Marion H., Robert E. Burrell, and Patricia L. Nadworny. "Evaluating antimicrobial efficacy of new commercially available silver dressings." *International Wound Journal* 7, no. 5 (2010): 394-405.

Chan, Marion Man-Ying. "Inhibition of tumor necrosis factor by curcumin, a phytochemical." *Biochemical pharmacology* 49, no. 11 (1995): 1551-1556.

Chang, Rachel Yoon Kyung, Theerthankar Das, Jim Manos, Elizabeth Kutter, Sandra Morales, and Hak-Kim Chan. "Bacteriophage PEV20 and ciprofloxacin combination treatment enhances removal of *Pseudomonas aeruginosa* biofilm isolated from cystic fibrosis and wound patients." *The AAPS Journal* 21, no. 3 (2019): 49.

Chatterjee, Arijit Kumar, Ruchira Chakraborty, and Tarakdas Basu. "Mechanism of antibacterial activity of copper nanoparticles." *Nanotechnology* 25, no. 13 (2014): 135101.

Chaw, K. C., M. Manimaran, and Francis EH Tay. "Role of silver ions in destabilization of intermolecular adhesion forces measured by atomic force microscopy in *Staphylococcus epidermidis* biofilms." *Antimicrobial agents and chemotherapy* 49, no. 12 (2005): 4853-4859.

Chou, Trong-Duo, Tz-Win Lee, Shao-Liang Chen, Yeou-Ming Tung, Nai-Tz Dai, Shyi-Gen Chen, Chiu-Hong Lee, Tim-Mo Chen, and Hsian-Jenn Wang. "The management of white phosphorus burns." *Burns* 27, no. 5 (2001): 492-497.

Cunningham, J. J., M. Leffell, and P. Harmatz. "Burn severity, copper dose, and plasma ceruloplasmin in burned children during total parenteral nutrition." *Nutrition (Burbank, Los Angeles County, Calif.)* 9, no. 4 (1993): 329-332.

DeLeon, Katrina, Fredrik Balldin, Chase Watters, Abdul Hamood, John Griswold, Sunil Sreedharan, and Kendra P. Rumbaugh. "Gallium maltolate treatment eradicates *Pseudomonas aeruginosa* infection in thermally injured mice." *Antimicrobial agents and chemotherapy* 53, no. 4 (2009): 1331-1337.

Dhivya, Selvaraj, Viswanadha Vijaya Padma, and Elango Santhini. "Wound dressings–a review." *BioMedicine* 5, no. 4 (2015).

Donlan, Rodney M. "Preventing biofilms of clinically relevant organisms using bacteriophage." *Trends in microbiology* 17, no. 2 (2009): 66-72.

Febré, Naldy, Viviana Silva, Andrea Báez, Humberto Palza, Katherine Delgado, Isabel Aburto, and Victor Silva. "Comportamiento antibacteriano de partículas de cobre frente a microorganismos obtenidos de úlceras crónicas infectadas y su relación con la resistencia a antimicrobianos de uso común." *Revista médica de Chile* 144, no. 12 (2016): 1523-1530.

Fleming, Irma D., Monika A. Krezalek, Natalia Belogortseva, Alexander Zaborin, Jennifer Defazio, Laxmipradha Chandrasekar, Luis A. Actis, Olga Zaborina, and John C. Alverdy. "Modeling *Acinetobacter baumannii* wound infections: The critical role of iron." *The journal of trauma and acute care surgery* 82, no. 3 (2017): 557.

Furfaro, Lucy L., Matthew S. Payne, and Barbara J. Chang. "Bacteriophage therapy: Clinical trials and regulatory hurdles." *Frontiers in cellular and infection microbiology* 8 (2018).

Gaddy, Jennifer A., Brock A. Arivett, Michael J. McConnell, Rafael López-Rojas, Jerónimo Pachón, and Luis A. Actis. "Role of acinetobactin-mediated iron acquisition functions in the interaction of *Acinetobacter baumannii* strain ATCC 19606T with human lung epithelial cells, *Galleria mellonella* caterpillars, and mice." *Infection and immunity* 80, no. 3 (2012): 1015-1024.

Gallant-Behm, Corrie L., Hua Q. Yin, Shijie Liu, John P. Heggers, Rita E. Langford, Merle E. Olson, David A. Hart, and Robert E. Burrell. "Comparison of in vitro disc diffusion and time kill-kinetic assays for the evaluation of antimicrobial wound dressing efficacy." *Wound repair and regeneration* 13, no. 4 (2005): 412-421.

Gallo, Richard L., and Teruaki Nakatsuji. "Microbial symbiosis with the innate immune defense system of the skin." *Journal of Investigative Dermatology* 131, no. 10 (2011): 1974-1980.

García-Quintanilla, Meritxell, Marina R. Pulido, Rafael López-Rojas, Jerónimo Pachón, and Michael J. McConnell. "Emerging therapies for multidrug *resistant Acinetobacter baumannii.*" *Trends in microbiology* 21, no. 3 (2013): 157-163.

Golbui Daghdari, Shabnam, Malahat Ahmadi, Habib Dastmalchi Saei, and Ali Asghar Tehrani. "The effect of ZnO nanoparticles on bacterial load of experimental infectious wounds contaminated with *Staphylococcus aureus* in mice." *Nanomedicine Journal* 4, no. 4 (2017): 232-236.

Gonzalez, Ana Cristina de Oliveira, Tila Fortuna Costa, Zilton de Araújo Andrade, and Alena Ribeiro Alves Peixoto Medrado. "Wound healing- A literature review." *Anais brasileiros de dermatologia* 91, no. 5 (2016): 614-620.

Gorbach, Sherwood L. "Antibiotic treatment of anaerobic infections." *Clinical infectious diseases* 18, no. Supplement_4 (1994): S305-S310.

Gottrup, Finn. "Prevention of surgical-wound infections." (2000): 202-204.

Grice, Elizabeth A., and Julia A. Segre. "The skin microbiome." *Nature Reviews Microbiology* 9, no. 4 (2011): 244.

Gueniche, A., B. Knaudt, E. Schuck, T. Volz, P. Bastien, R. Martin, M. Röcken, L. Breton, and T. Biedermann. "Effects of nonpathogenic gram-negative bacterium *Vitreoscilla filiformis* lysate on atopic dermatitis: a prospective, randomized, double-blind, placebo-controlled clinical study." *British Journal of Dermatology* 159, no. 6 (2008): 1357-1363.

Gupta, Pooja, Hari Shankar Singh, Vijay K. Shukla, Gopal Nath, and Satyanam Kumar Bhartiya. "Bacteriophage therapy of chronic nonhealing wound: Clinical study." *The international journal of lower extremity wounds* (2019): 1534734619835115.

Halstead, Fenella D., Maryam Rauf, Amy Bamford, Christopher M. Wearn, Jonathan RB Bishop, Rebecca Burt, Adam P. Fraise, Naiem S. Moiemen, Beryl A. Oppenheim, and Mark A. Webber. "Antimicrobial dressings: comparison of the ability of a panel of dressings to prevent biofilm formation by key burn wound pathogens." *Burns* 41, no. 8 (2015): 1683-1694.

Han, George, and Roger Ceilley. "Chronic wound healing: a review of current management and treatments." *Advances in therapy* 34, no. 3 (2017): 599-610.

Heal, Clare F., Jennifer L. Banks, Phoebe D. Lepper, Evangelos Kontopantelis, and Mieke L. van Driel. "Topical antibiotics for preventing surgical site infection in wounds healing by primary intention." *Cochrane Database of Systematic Reviews* 11 (2016).

Hegerova, Dagmar, Cihalova Kristyna, Kopel Pavel, Adam Vojtech, and Kizek Rene. "Selenium nanoparticles and evaluation of their antimicrobial activity on bacterial isolates obtained from clinical specimens." *Nanocon. Oct 14th–16th* (2015).

Hernandez, Robert. "The use of systemic antibiotics in the treatment of chronic wounds." *Dermatologic therapy* 19, no. 6 (2006): 326-337.

Hersh, Adam L., Henry F. Chambers, Judith H. Maselli, and Ralph Gonzales. "National trends in ambulatory visits and antibiotic prescribing for skin and soft-tissue infections." *Archives of internal medicine* 168, no. 14 (2008): 1585-1591.

Hussein, Saba Zuhair, Kamaruddin Mohd Yusoff, Suzana Makpol, Mohd Yusof, and Yasmin Anum. "Gelam honey inhibits the production of proinflammatory, mediators NO, PGE2, TNF-α, and IL-6 in carrageenan-induced acute paw edema in rats." *Evidence-Based Complementary and Alternative Medicine* (2012).

James, Garth A., Ellen Swogger, Randall Wolcott, Elinor Delancey Pulcini, Patrick Secor, Jennifer Sestrich, John W. Costerton, and Philip S. Stewart. "Biofilms in chronic wounds." *Wound Repair and regeneration* 16, no. 1 (2008): 37-44.

Jault, Patrick, Thomas Leclerc, Serge Jennes, Jean Paul Pirnay, Yok-Ai Que, Gregory Resch, Anne Françoise Rousseau et al. "Efficacy and tolerability of a cocktail of bacteriophages to treat burn wounds infected by *Pseudomonas aeruginosa* (PhagoBurn): A randomised, controlled, double-blind phase 1/2 trial." *The Lancet Infectious Diseases* 19, no. 1 (2019): 35-45.

Jones, Vanessa, Joseph E. Grey, and Keith G. Harding. "Wound dressings." *Bmj* 332, no. 7544 (2006): 777-780.

K Chan, Benjamin, and Stephen T Abedon. "Bacteriophages and their enzymes in biofilm control." *Current pharmaceutical design* 21, no. 1 (2015): 85-99.

Kadam, Snehal, Saptarsi Shai, Aditi Shahane, and Karishma S. Kaushik. "Recent advances in non-conventional antimicrobial approaches for chronic wound biofilms: have we found the 'chink in the armor'?" *Biomedicines* 7, no. 2 (2019): 35.

Kalia, Vipin Chandra. "Quorum sensing inhibitors: an overview." *Biotechnology advances* 31, no. 2 (2013): 224-245.

Kao, Ming-Shan, Stephen Huang, Wei-Lin Chang, Ming-Fa Hsieh, Chun-Jen Huang, Richard L. Gallo, and Chun-Ming Huang. "Microbiome precision editing: Using PEG as a selective fermentation initiator against methicillin-resistant *Staphylococcus aureus.*" *Biotechnology journal* 12, no. 4 (2017).

Karumathil, Deepti P., Meera Surendran Nair, James Gaffney, Anup Kollanoor-Johny, and Kumar Venkitanarayanan. "Trans-Cinnamaldehyde and eugenol Increase *Acinetobacter baumannii* sensitivity to beta-lactam antibiotics." *Frontiers in microbiology* 9 (2018).

Karumathil, Deepti P., Meera Surendran-Nair, and Kumar Venki-tanarayanan. "Efficacy of trans-cinnamaldehyde and eugenol in reducing *Acinetobacter baumannii* adhesion to and invasion of human keratinocytes and controlling wound infection *in vitro.*" *Phytotherapy Research* 30, no. 12 (2016): 2053-2059.

Kaufman, Kathryn L., F. A. Mann, Dae Young Kim, Suhwon Lee, and Hun-Young Yoon. "Evaluation of the effects of topical zinc gluconate in wound healing." *Veterinary surgery* 43, no. 8 (2014): 972-982.

Kong, Heidi H. "Skin microbiome: genomics-based insights into the diversity and role of skin microbes." *Trends in molecular medicine* 17, no. 6 (2011): 320-328.

Kornblatt, Allison Paige, Vincenzo Giuseppe Nicoletti, and Alessio Travaglia. "The neglected role of copper ions in wound healing." *Journal of inorganic biochemistry* 161 (2016): 1-8.

Lansdown, Alan BG, Ursula Mirastschijski, Nicky Stubbs, Elizabeth Scanlon, and Magnus S. Ågren. "Zinc in wound healing: theoretical, experimental, and clinical aspects." *Wound repair and regeneration* 15, no. 1 (2007): 2-16.

Lau, Patrck. *The efficacy of zinc and manganese in controlling methicillin-resistant Staphylococcus aureus wound infections in vitro.* OpenCommons@UConn (Honors scholar theses). Available online: https://opencommons.uconn.edu/srhonors_theses/508/

Leaper, David J. "Prophylactic and therapeutic role of antibiotics in wound care." *The American journal of surgery* 167, no. 1 (1994): S15-S20.

Lemire, Joseph A., Joe J. Harrison, and Raymond J. Turner. "Antimicrobial activity of metals: mechanisms, molecular targets and applications." *Nature Reviews Microbiology* 11, no. 6 (2013): 371.

Li, Ying, Jen Hsin, Lingyun Zhao, Yiwen Cheng, Weina Shang, Kerwyn Casey Huang, Hong-Wei Wang, and Sheng Ye. "FtsZ protofilaments use a hinge-opening mechanism for constrictive force generation." *Science* 341, no. 6144 (2013): 392-395.

Liakos, Ioannis, L. Rizzello, Hadi Hajiali, Virgilio Brunetti, Riccardo Carzino, P. P. Pompa, Athanassia Athanassiou, and Elisa Mele. "Fibrous wound dressings encapsulating essential oils as natural antimicrobial agents." *Journal of Materials Chemistry B* 3, no. 8 (2015): 1583-1589.

Liu, Su-Hsun, Yhu-Chering Huang, Leslie Y. Chen, Shu-Chuan Yu, Hsiao-Yun Yu, and Shiow-Shuh Chuang. "The skin microbiome of wound scars and unaffected skin in patients with moderate to severe burns in the subacute phase." *Wound Repair and Regeneration* 26, no. 2 (2018): 182-191.

Mackowiak, Philip A. "The normal microbial flora." *New England Journal of Medicine* 307, no. 2 (1982): 83-93.

Majtan, Juraj, Jana Bohova, Rocio Garcia-Villalba, Francisco A. Tomas-Barberan, Zuzana Madakova, Tomas Majtan, Viktor Majtan, and Jaroslav Klaudiny. "Fir honeydew honey flavonoids inhibit TNF-α-induced MMP-9 expression in human keratinocytes: a new action of honey in wound healing." *Archives of dermatological research* 305, no. 7 (2013): 619-627.

Majtan, Juraj. "Honey: an immunomodulator in wound healing." *Wound Repair and Regeneration* 22, no. 2 (2014): 187-192.

Mendes, João J., Clara Leandro, Sofia Corte-Real, Raquel Barbosa, Patrícia Cavaco-Silva, José Melo-Cristino, Andrzej Górski, and Miguel Garcia. "Wound healing potential of topical bacteriophage therapy on diabetic cutaneous wounds." *Wound Repair and Regeneration* 21, no. 4 (2013): 595-603.

Milho, C., M. Andrade, D. Vilas Boas, Diana Alves, and Sanna Sillankorva. "Antimicrobial assessment of phage therapy using a porcine model of biofilm infection." *International journal of pharmaceutics* 557 (2019): 112-123.

Mohandas, Annapoorna, S. Deepthi, Raja Biswas, and R. Jayakumar. "Chitosan based metallic nanocomposite scaffolds as antimicrobial wound dressings." *Bioactive materials* 3, no. 3 (2018): 267-277.

Molan, Peter C. "Potential of honey in the treatment of wounds and burns." *American journal of clinical dermatology* 2, no. 1 (2001): 13-19.

Nair, Divek VT, and Anup Kollanoor Johny. "Food grade Pimenta leaf essential oil reduces the attachment *of Salmonella enterica* Heidelberg (2011 ground turkey outbreak isolate) on to turkey skin." *Frontiers in microbiology* 8 (2017): 2328.

Nakatsuji, Teruaki, Tiffany H. Chen, Aimee M. Two, Kimberly A. Chun, Saisindhu Narala, Raif S. Geha, Tissa R. Hata, and Richard L. Gallo. "*Staphylococcus aureus* exploits epidermal barrier defects in atopic dermatitis to trigger cytokine expression." *Journal of Investigative Dermatology* 136, no. 11 (2016): 2192-2200.

Negut, Irina, Valentina Grumezescu, and Alexandru Grumezescu. "Treatment strategies for infected wounds." *Molecules* 23, no. 9 (2018): 2392.

Nichols, Ronald Lee. "Preventing surgical site infections: a surgeon's perspective." *Emerging infectious diseases* 7, no. 2 (2001): 220.

Ozay, Yusuf, Sevda Guzel, Ibrahim Halil Erdogdu, Zuhal Yildirim, Burcin Pehlivanoglu, Bilge Aydın Turk, and Sinan Darcan. "Evaluation of the wound healing properties of luteolin ointments on excision and incision wound models in diabetic and non-diabetic rats." *Records of Natural Products*12, no. 4 (2018).

Percival, Steven L., Sara M. McCarty, and Benjamin Lipsky. "Biofilms and wounds: an overview of the evidence." *Advances in Wound Care* 4, no. 7 (2015): 373-381.

Percival, Steven, and Keith Cutting. *Microbiology of wounds.* CRC press, 2010.

Plichta, Jennifer K., Xiang Gao, Huaiying Lin, Qunfeng Dong, Evelyn Toh, David E. Nelson, Richard L. Gamelli, Elizabeth A. Grice, and Katherine A. Radek. "Cutaneous burn injury promotes shifts in the bacterial microbiome in autologous donor skin: implications for skin grafting outcomes." *Shock (Augusta, Ga.)* 48, no. 4 (2017): 441-448.

Poutahidis, Theofilos, Sean M. Kearney, Tatiana Levkovich, Peimin Qi, Bernard J. Varian, Jessica R. Lakritz, Yassin M. Ibrahim, Antonis Chatzigiagkos, Eric J. Alm, and Susan E. Erdman. "Microbial symbionts accelerate wound healing via the neuropeptide hormone oxytocin." *PloS one* 8, no. 10 (2013).

Price, Philip B. "The bacteriology of normal skin; a new quantitative test applied to a study of the bacterial flora and the disinfectant action of mechanical cleansing." *The journal of infectious diseases* (1938): 301-318.

Raghupathi, Krishna R., Ranjit T. Koodali, and Adhar C. Manna. "Size-dependent bacterial growth inhibition and mechanism of antibacterial activity of zinc oxide nanoparticles." *Langmuir* 27, no. 7 (2011): 4020-4028.

Raguvaran, R., Anju Manuja, and Balvinder Kumar Manuja. "Zinc oxide nanoparticles: opportunities and challenges in veterinary sciences." *Immunome Research* 11, no. 2 (2015): 1.

Rai, Dipti, Jay Kumar Singh, Nilanjan Roy, and Dulal Panda. "Curcumin inhibits FtsZ assembly: an attractive mechanism for its antibacterial activity." *Biochemical Journal* 410, no. 1 (2008): 147-155.

Reddy, Kongara M., Kevin Feris, Jason Bell, Denise G. Wingett, Cory Hanley, and Alex Punnoose. "Selective toxicity of zinc oxide nanoparticles to prokaryotic and eukaryotic systems." *Applied physics letters* 90, no. 21 (2007): 213902.

Rose, Thomas, Gilbert Verbeken, Daniel De Vos, Maya Merabishvili, Mario Vaneechoutte, Rob Lavigne, Serge Jennes, Martin Zizi, and Jean-Paul Pirnay. "Experimental phage therapy of burn wound infection: difficult first steps." *International journal of burns and trauma* 4, no. 2 (2014): 66.

Schierle, Clark F., Mauricio De la Garza, Thomas A. Mustoe, and Robert D. Galiano. "Staphylococcal biofilms impair wound healing by delaying reepithelialization in a murine cutaneous wound model." *Wound Repair and Regeneration* 17, no. 3 (2009): 354-359.

Schmidt, Cleber A., Renato Murillo, Torsten Bruhn, Gerhard Bringmann, Marcia Goettert, Berta Heinzmann, Volker Brecht, Stefan A. Laufer, and Irmgard Merfort. "Catechin derivatives from *Parapiptadenia rigida* with *in vitro* wound-healing properties." *Journal of natural Products* 73, no. 12 (2010): 2035-2041.

Schultz, Gregory S., R. Gary Sibbald, Vincent Falanga, Elizabeth A. Ayello, Caroline Dowsett, Keith Harding, Marco Romanelli, Michael C. Stacey, Luc Teot, and Wolfgang Vanscheidt. "Wound bed preparation: a systematic approach to wound management." *Wound repair and regeneration* 11 (2003): S1-S28.

Schwarz, Agatha, Anika Bruhs, and Thomas Schwarz. "The short-chain fatty acid sodium butyrate functions as a regulator of the skin immune system." *Journal of Investigative Dermatology* 137, no. 4 (2017): 855-864.

Scutera, Sara, Mario Zucca, and Dianella Savoia. "Novel approaches for the design and discovery of quorum-sensing inhibitors." *Expert Opinion on Drug Discovery* 9, no. 4 (2014): 353-366.

Seil, Justin T., and Thomas J. Webster. "Antimicrobial applications of nanotechnology: methods and literature." *International journal of nanomedicine* 7 (2012): 2767.

Semeniuc, Cristina Anamaria, Carmen Rodica Pop, and Ancuţa Mihaela Rotar. "Antibacterial activity and interactions of plant essential oil combinations against Gram-positive and Gram-negative bacteria." *journal of food and drug analysis* 25, no. 2 (2017): 403-408.

Sen, Chandan K., Gayle M. Gordillo, Sashwati Roy, Robert Kirsner, Lynn Lambert, Thomas K. Hunt, Finn Gottrup, Geoffrey C. Gurtner, and Michael T. Longaker. "Human skin wounds: a major and snowballing threat to public health and the economy." *Wound repair and regeneration* 17, no. 6 (2009): 763-771.

Sen, Chandan K., Savita Khanna, Mika Venojarvi, Prashant Trikha, E. Christopher Ellison, Thomas K. Hunt, and Sashwati Roy. "Copper-induced vascular endothelial growth factor expression and wound healing." *American Journal of Physiology-Heart and Circulatory Physiology* 282, no. 5 (2002): H1821-H1827.

Sengupta, Aniruddha, Ulrike F. Lichti, Bradley A. Carlson, Andrew O. Ryscavage, Vadim N. Gladyshev, Stuart H. Yuspa, and Dolph L. Hatfield. "Selenoproteins are essential for proper keratinocyte function and skin development." *PloS one* 5, no. 8 (2010): e12249.

Seth, Akhil K., Matthew R. Geringer, Khang T. Nguyen, Sonya P. Agnew, Zari Dumanian, Robert D. Galiano, Kai P. Leung, Thomas A. Mustoe, and Seok J. Hong. "Bacteriophage therapy for *Staphylococcus aureus* biofilm–infected wounds: a new approach to chronic wound care." *Plastic and reconstructive surgery* 131, no. 2 (2013): 225-234.

Shah, Ahmed, and Saeid Amini-Nik. "The role of phytochemicals in the inflammatory phase of wound healing." *International journal of molecular sciences* 18, no. 5 (2017): 1068.

Sienkiewicz, Monika, Anna Głowacka, Edward Kowalczyk, Anna Wiktorowska-Owczarek, Marta Jóźwiak-Bębenista, and Monika Łysakowska. "The biological activities of cinnamon, geranium and lavender essential oils." *Molecules* 19, no. 12 (2014): 20929-20940.

Singer, Adam J., and Richard AF Clark. "Cutaneous wound healing." *New England journal of medicine* 341, no. 10 (1999): 738-746.

Singh, Sanjaya, and Bharat B. Aggarwal. "Activation of transcription factor NF-κB is suppressed by curcumin (diferuloylmethane)." *Journal of Biological Chemistry* 270, no. 42 (1995): 24995-25000.

Somerville, Dorothy A., and W. C. Noble. "Microcolony size of microbes on human skin." *Journal of medical microbiology* 6, no. 3 (1973): 323-328.

Somerville-Millar, Dorothy A., and W. C. Noble. "Resident and transient bacteria of the skin." *Journal of cutaneous pathology* 1, no. 6 (1974): 260-264.

Song, Joon Young, Sae Yoon Kee, In Sook Hwang, Yu Bin Seo, Hye Won Jeong, Woo Joo Kim, and Hee Jin Cheong. "*In vitro* activities of carbapenem/sulbactam combination, colistin, colistin/rifampicin combination and tigecycline against carbapenem-resistant *Acineto-bacter baumannii*." *Journal of antimicrobial chemotherapy* 60, no. 2 (2007): 317-322.

Surendran Nair, Meera, Yanyan Liu, and Kumar Venkitanarayanan. "Selenium increases sensitivity of multi-drug resistant *Acinetobacter baumannii* wound isolates to antibiotics through synergistic interactions." 2016 *American Society for Microbiology Microbe Annual Meeting Abstract.*

Surendran Nair, Meera, Patrick Lau, Yanyan Liu, and Kumar Venkitanarayanan. "Efficacy of selenium in controlling *Acinetobacter baumannii* associated wound infections." *Wound Medicine* (2019) : 100165.

Tran, Ngoc Quyen, Yoon Ki Joung, Eugene Lih, and Ki Dong Park. "*In situ* forming and rutin-releasing chitosan hydrogels as injectable dressings for dermal wound healing." *Biomacromolecules* 12, no. 8 (2011): 2872-2880.

Tran, Phat, Saurabh Patel, Abdul Hamood, Tyler Enos, Thomas Mosley, Courtney Jarvis, Akash Desai, Pamela Lin, and Ted Reid. "A novel organo-selenium bandage that inhibits biofilm development in a wound by Gram-positive and Gram-negative wound pathogens." *Antibiotics* 3, no. 3 (2014): 435-449.

Valdez, J. C., M. C. Peral, M. Rachid, M. Santana, and G. Perdigon. "Interference of *Lactobacillus plantarum* with *Pseudomonas aeruginosa in vitro* and in infected burns: the potential use of probiotics in wound treatment." *Clinical microbiology and infection* 11, no. 6 (2005): 472-479.

Williams, Michael R., and Richard L. Gallo. "The role of the skin microbiome in atopic dermatitis." *Current allergy and asthma reports* 15, no. 11 (2015): 65.

Williamson, Deborah A., Glen P. Carter, and Benjamin P. Howden. "Current and emerging topical antibacterials and antiseptics: agents, action, and resistance patterns." *Clinical microbiology reviews* 30, no. 3 (2017): 827-860.

Wolcott, Randall D., John D. Hanson, Eric J. Rees, Lawrence D. Koenig, Caleb D. Phillips, Richard A. Wolcott, Stephen B. Cox, and Jennifer S. White. "Analysis of the chronic wound microbiota of 2,963 patients by 16S rDNA pyrosequencing." *Wound Repair and Regeneration* 24, no. 1 (2016): 163-174.

Yah, Clarence S., and Geoffrey S. Simate. "Nanoparticles as potential new generation broad spectrum antimicrobial agents." *DARU Journal of Pharmaceutical Sciences* 23, no. 1 (2015): 43.

You, Chuangang, Qiong Li, Xingang Wang, Pan Wu, Jon Kee Ho, Ronghua Jin, Liping Zhang, Huawei Shao, and Chunmao Han. "Silver nanoparticle loaded collagen/chitosan scaffolds promote wound healing via regulating fibroblast migration and macrophage activation." *Scientific reports* 7, no. 1 (2017): 10489.

Zeeuwen, Patrick LJM, Michiel Kleerebezem, Harro M. Timmerman, and Joost Schalkwijk. "Microbiome and skin diseases." *Current opinion in allergy and clinical immunology* 13, no. 5 (2013): 514-520.

In: A Closer Look at Wound Infections ...   ISBN: 978-1-53616-816-7
Editor: Joseph E. Keel   © 2020 Nova Science Publishers, Inc.

Chapter 3

THE ROLE OF ESTROGENIC SUBSTANCES IN REGULATIONS OF BIOLOGICAL PROCESSES INVOLVED INTO WOUND HEALING

Luigi Filocamo[*], Luisa Maria Migneco,
Francesca Ceccacci and Francesca Leonelli
[1]Department of Biochemical Science "A. Rossi Fanelli,"
University "La Sapienza," Rome, Italy
[2]Department of Chemistry, University "La Sapienza," Rome, Italy
[3]Institute for Biological Systems - CNR,
Support organizational unit, "La Sapienza," Rome, Italy
[4]Department of Environmental Biology,
University "La Sapienza," Rome, Italy

ABSTRACT

Wound healing is a physiological process that involves several successive and often overlapping phases that lead to the restoration of the integrity of the skin after an injury, accident or surgery: haemostasis and

[*] Corresponding Author's E-mail: luigi.filocamo@uniroma1.it.

inflammation, proliferation and remodeling. The interruption or slowing down of these processes can cause abnormal or impaired wound healing. There are now numerous data and clinical studies that highlight the role of estrogens on normal cutaneous homeostasis and wound healing. In postmenopausal women, for example, the reduced rate of wound healing processes has been clearly related to estrogen deficiency, especially in relation to inflammation and re-granulation, while treatment with exogenous estrogens can reverse these effects. We report here the complex role of estrogens and estrogenic derivatives in wound healing process, with a focus on their therapeutic use, and which strategies have been explored to find substances with poor systemic effects.

Keywords: wound healing, estrogen, estrogen receptor, soft drugs, SERM, phytoestrogens

WOUND HEALING SEQUENCE OF EVENTS

Wound healing is a complex multistage process extensively investigated over the years (Figure 1). Diverse major events correlated with healing have been discussed in the literature (Singer and Clark 1999; Gurtner et al. 2008; Kirsner and Eaglstein 1993).

The process involves an array of cells and events, starting with blood clotting and inflammation, followed by proliferation and migration of dermal and epidermal cells, ending with matrix synthesis to take over the wound gap and restore tissue integrity and homeostasis (Hackam and Ford 2002; Harding, Moore, and Phillips 2005). The last phase consists of tissue remodeling and differentiation to completely restore the skin functionality and reparair skin tissue (Diegelmann and Evans 2004; Hynes 2009; Hackam and Ford 2002). This sequence of events, especially during the first phases, is regulated by a plethora of cellular mediators comprising eicosanoids, cytokines, nitric oxide, and various growth factors. Interleukin-1 (IL-1) is stored in large amounts in the epidermis of intact skin and is the first mediator that warns surrounding cells of damage to the integrity of the tissue (Bochner et al. 1990; Corsini et al. 1998; Freedberg et al. 2001; Murphy, Robert, and Kupper 2000). The activation of the clotting cascade induces haemostasis by activation, adhesion and aggregation of platelets, and the resulting clot provides a matrix influx of inflammatory cells. Subsequently, the alpha granules, that are a cellular component of platelets, secrete various growth factors: epidermal growth factor (EGF), platelet-derived growth factor (PDGF), insulin-like growth factors (IGFs) and transforming growth factor-β (TGF-β), which are the leading mediator of the proliferation phase. (Barrientos et al. 2008; Lawrence 1998; Nurden et al. 2008). PDGF, together with proinflammatory cytokines such as IL-1, has the task of attracting neutrophils and, subsequently, macrophages, endothelial cells and fibroblasts (Barrientos et al. 2008; Velnar, Bailey, and Smrkolj 2009; Glaros, Larsen, and Li 2009). Another growth factor released by the platelets, the vascular endothelial growth factor (VEGF), triggers the proliferation of endothelial cells, and the fibroblast growth factor (FGF) eventually promotes angiogenesis (Tassi et al. 2011; Bao et al. 2009). Neovascularization is essential for the synthesis, deposition and organization of a new extracellular matrix (ECM). Dynamic interactions between growth factors and ECM are integral to wound healing (Schultz and Wysocki 2009). FGF, TGF-β, and PDGFs derived from macrophages cause fibroblast infiltration and phenotypic conversion into myofibroblasts bearing α-smooth muscle actin (αSMA) (Evans et al. 2003; Serini et al. 1998). The function of myofibroblasts is to facilitate wound healing by combining the extracellular matrix (ECM)–synthesizing features of fibroblasts with cytoskeletal characteristics of contractile smooth muscle cells (Hinz et al. 2012). To complete the formation of the matrix and begin the remodeling phase it is necessary to replace the granulation tissue with a structure of collagen and elastin fibers and finally revascularize the tissue. This remodeling process begins two or three weeks after the injury and lasts for a year or more (Buckley et al. 2001; Barrientos et al. 2008). Finally, most endothelial cells, along with macrophages and fibroblasts, undergo apoptosis, and leave a mass of a few cells, which consist mainly of collagen and other extracellular matrix proteins, and the final product of this process is scar tissue (Monaco and Lawrence 2003).

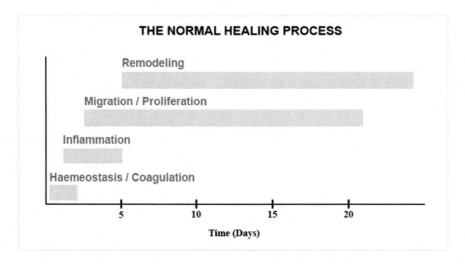

Figure 1. The normal healing process: overlapping healing phases (simplified). After injury, platelet aggregation and recruitment of complement factors at the wound site stimulate inflammation, cell migration and proliferation, leading to matrix synthesis, contraction, angiogenesis and ultimately remodeling.

ESTROGEN RECEPTORS

The three main natural estrogen hormones are estrone (E1), estradiol (E2) and estriol (E3) (Figure 2). Estrogens are normally present at lower levels than androgens in both men and women (Burger 2002), and although estrogen levels are significantly lower in males than females, they also have important physiological roles in males (Lombardi et al. 2001).

Like all steroid hormones, estrogens can easily diffuse through the cell membrane and interact with specific receptors through both genomic and non-genomic signaling mechanisms. Estrogen genomic signaling is the predominant mechanism and involves binding of two nuclear receptors for estrogens (ER) named ER-α and ER-β, encoded respectively by ESR1 and ESR2 genes. ERs have different molecular weights, ERα consist of 595 and ERβ of 530 amino acids (Kumar et al. 2011). The receptors structure includes six domains (Figure 3). The A/B domains are involved in transcriptional activation and contain the transcriptional regulatory domain (constitutively active amino-terminal domain, AF-1), the C domain contains the conserved zinc finger DNA binding domain (estrogen-responsive element, ERE). The following D domain, also called hinge region, contains nuclear localization signals (NLSs) and makes the protein flexible between the DNA-binding domain and the ligand-binding domain (LBD). The domain E contains the ligands pocket (LBD), along with the activator factor-2 (AF-2), which mediates a wide range of functional responses, and domain F is the carboxy-terminal of the ERs (Hewitt and Korach 2018).

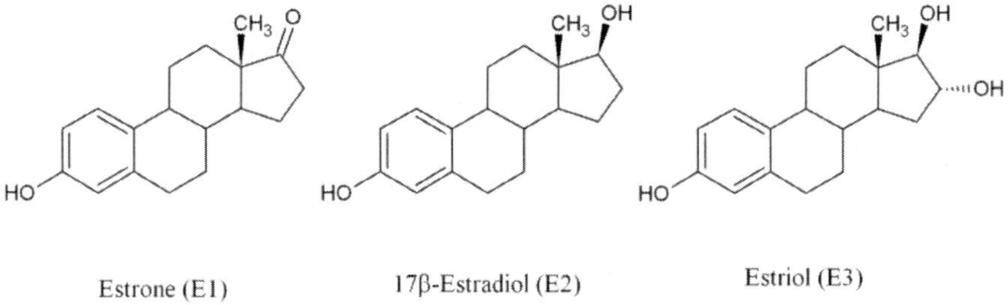

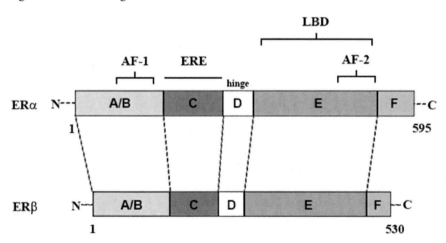

Figure 2. Natural estrogen hormones.

Figure 3. Structure of estrogen receptors. AF-1 (activator factor-1), ERE (estrogen responsive element), LBD (ligand binding domain), AF-2 (activator factor-2).

The estrogen binding to their nuclear receptors causes dissociation from the receptors inhibitory protein and homo- or hetero-dimerization to form a complex that acts as a transcription factor interacting with gene promoters to trigger up- or down-regulation of target genes. Others genomic mechanisms involving indirect binding to other existing transcription factors (tethering), and ligand-independent receptor activation have been characterized (Hamilton et al. 2017).

There is ample evidence of the presence of ERs in multiple cell types involved in the wound healing process, such as inflammatory cells, and vascular endothelial cells, suggesting that estrogen could have a role in the modulation of multiple aspects in wound healing (Trenti et al. 2018; Gulshan, McCruden, and Stimson 1990). ER-α and ER-β are the two predominant forms of ERs identified in the skin and bind to estradiol with similar affinity. (Bai and Gust 2009; Pelletier and Ren 2004). The expression of the two estrogen receptors is markedly different in human skin derived from distinct anatomical sites such as scalp, breast and abdomen. For example, unlike breast skin, which mainly expresses ER-α, scalp predominantly expresses ER-β (Stevenson and Thornton 2007). ER-β is most expressed in the epidermis, dermal fibroblasts, blood vessels, and hair follicles of human scalp skin (Thornton et al. 2003), while the expression of ER-α is inducted in keratinocytes of neonatal skin (Verdier-Sevrain et al. 2004).

Non-genomic estrogenic signaling is less well understood, but generally occurs considerably faster than genomic signaling and proceeds via cytosolic pathways involving classical second messengers (Manavathi and Kumar 2006). Membrane-associated full-length ER-α and two truncated isoforms, ER-α 46 kDa and ER-α 36 kDa, exist that are at least in part responsible for such signaling (Razandi et al. 2004; Chen et al. 1999; Figtree et al. 2003; Li, Haynes, and Bender 2003; Chambliss et al. 2010; Kang et al. 2010). However, much less information is available regarding non-genomic actions of ER-β (Chambliss et al. 2002; Abrahám et al. 2003; Moro et al. 2005).

An orphan G-protein coupled receptor (GPCR), GPR30, was identified in 2005 as an estrogen-binding intracellular membrane GPCR (Prossnitz et al. 2008; Revankar et al. 2005; Thomas et al. 2005) after it had been previously shown that its expression was required for rapid cellular responses to 17β-estradiol (E2) (Maggiolini et al. 2004; Filardo et al. 2000; Filardo and Thomas 2012). This receptor is now included in the official GPCR nomenclature and was designated G protein-coupled estrogen (GPER) by the International Union of Pharmacology in 2007 (Alexander, Mathie, and Peters 2011). Some experimental evidence suggests that E2 may enhance the proliferation and functions of human keratinocytes via GPER (Kanda and Watanabe 2004b, 2004a; Verdier-Sevrain et al. 2004).

ESTROGENS AND WOUND HEALING

The effects of estrogen on wound healing processes have been known since the late 1940s (Sjövall 1947; Sjostedt 1953). Since then, a large number of studies, especially on animal models, has provided further evidence of the importance of the role of estrogen in wound healing and has provided more information on the mechanisms underlying estrogen activity. The most widely used animal model for testing the effect of estrogenic substances on wound healing is the (OVX) ovariectomized female mice, while for clinical studies variations in wound healing rate and quality are observed in postmenopausal women and aged humans. There is ample evidence that estrogen replacement accelerates cutaneous healing in ovariectomized (OVX) female mice and rats (Wilkinson and Hardman 2017; Mukai et al. 2016a; Mukai et al. 2016b; Ashcroft et al. 1997, 2003; Emmerson et al. 2010; Hardman et al. 2008), while estrogen role in males remains to be well established. Acceleration of wound healing in young OVX female mice and old male mice after systemic treatment with sex steroid precursor dehydroepiandrosterone (DHEA) was observed, and this result was attributed to the local conversion of DHEA to estrogen (Mills et al. 2005). There are important differences in the mechanisms that control repairs in males and females. The androgens' detrimental effects to healing are confirmed by the observation that testosterone metabolite 5α-dihydrotestosterone (DHT) retards repair in male rats (Gilliver et al. 2009), and gonadectomy (GDX) or androgen receptor blockade improves healing in male rodents (Gilliver, Wu, and Ashcroft 2003; Ashcroft and Mills 2002; Gilliver et al. 2006), while ovariectomy worsens healing in females presumably because of the lack of estrogen regulation of the proinflammatory and pleiotropic cytokine macrophage migration inhibitory factor of (MIF) (Gilliver et al. 2008). MIF is widely expressed during tissue repair, however, its precise function in wound healing and wound cell physiology is still to be cleared (Gilliver et al. 2011). The link between MIF and sex steroids in the context of wound healing is increasingly evident; in fact, wound levels of MIF (Ashcroft et al. 2003), intracellular MIF-signaling mediator CSN5 (Gilliver et al. 2008), and MIF receptor CD74 (Emmerson et al. 2010; Hardman et al. 2008) are significantly increased in OVX mice. Furthermore, wound MIF levels are considerably increased in postmenopausal women and decrease by hormone replacement therapy (HRT) (Hardman et al. 2005). MIF level increase, observed in wounds of OVX mice, is blocked by systemic administration of estrogen or selective estrogen receptor modulators (SERMs) tamoxifen, raloxifene (Hardman et al. 2008) or genistein (Emmerson et al. 2010), or by local administration of E2 derivatives (Brufani et al. 2009, 2017). Notwithstanding intensive research, there is still no general consensus as to MIF primary function in cutaneous wound healing, however, several studies supply convincing evidence that MIF impairs healing. In MIF knockout mice (KO) gonadectomy still improves healing in males but does not have explicit effects on female mice, and the local administration of MIF worsens repair on OVX, KO females, but not on GDX, KO males (Gilliver et al. 2008). In a further study, the lack of efficacy of E2 local treatment on wound healing was reiterated again. Fifty-six male mice aged 7 weeks were divided into 4 groups: sham-operated (sham), castrated (CSX), sham-operated treated with E2 (sham + E), and CSX treated with E2 (CSX + E). During the wound healing process E2 reduced macrophages number in inflammatory phase without significant differences between the groups in the reduction of scarring and re-epithelialization of wounds (Nakajima et al. 2013).

While the effects of estrogen administration lead to conflicting results in male wound healing processes, the beneficial effects of local or systemic administration in females are widely documented. The finding of a link between the physiological changes following menopause and delayed healing of acute wounds in elderly women (Ashcroft et al. 1997) induced to explore further the roles of estrogens in wound inflammation. Acceleration of healing in elderly females by topically-applied estradiol was accompanied by an early decrease in wound neutrophil numbers due to direct inhibition of chemotaxis and attenuated expression of the cell adhesion molecule L-selectin. The suppression of neutrophil accumulation has, as a consequence, a reduction of neutrophil elastase activity and fibronectin degradation. The consequent increment in local fibronectin amplifies the inflow of fibroblasts and the deposition of collagen. Furthermore, since elastase activates matrix metalloproteinases, a reduced activity of elastase would dramatically reduce collagen degradation, encouraging healing. The observed increase in wound contraction would therefore be due to a combination of contraction mediated by myofibroblasts and re-epithelialization (Ashcroft et al. 1999). Also, estrogen replacement by SERM or estradiol derivatives in rodents markedly reverses the increase in wound inflammation that occurs as a consequence of ovariectomy, decreasing the overall local number of neutrophils (Hardman et al. 2008; Brufani et al. 2009, 2017), CD163-positive leukocytes and macrophages activated in a classical manner, while increasing the alternatively-activated macrophage population, and reducing wound levels of IL-6, tumor necrosis factor (TNF-α) and macrophage migration inhibitory factor (MIF), as well as the putative MIF receptor CD74 (Schultz and Wysocki 2009; Ashcroft et al. 1999; Leng et al. 2003; Brufani et al. 2009, 2017). The connection between estrogens and wound inflammation is reinforced by genetic studies that established a correlation between polymorphisms in the ESR2 gene and incidence of venous ulceration, a condition characterized by unresolved inflammation (Ashworth et al. 2005, 2008).

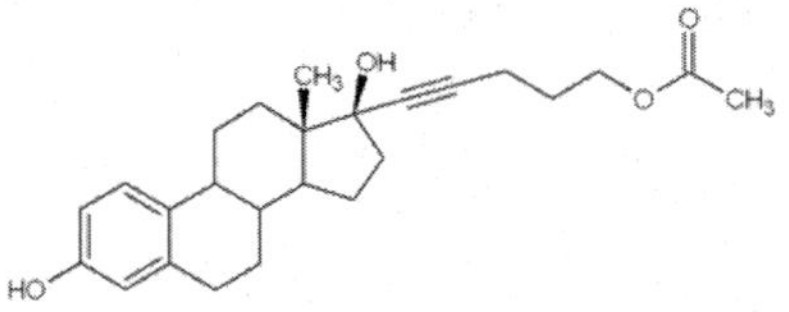

Figure 4. Compounds 1 and 2 display a significant regenerative and anti-inflammatory activity without systemic effects after local administration in OVX mice.

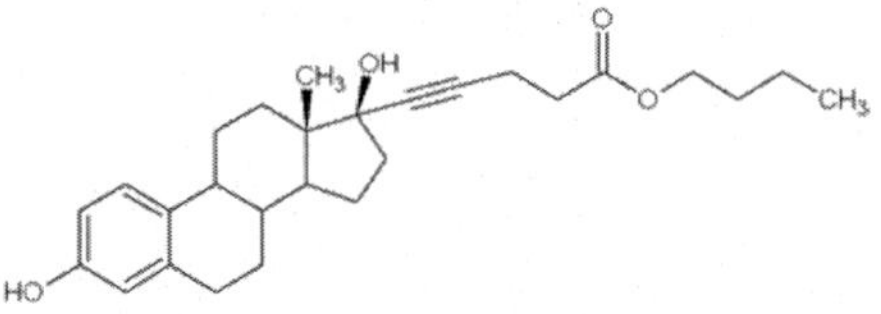

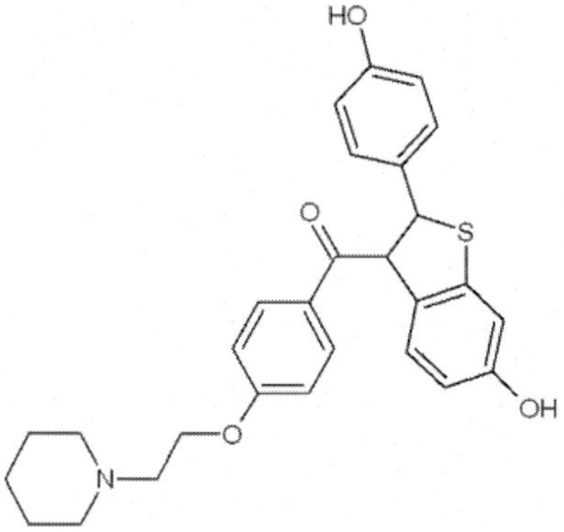

Raloxifene

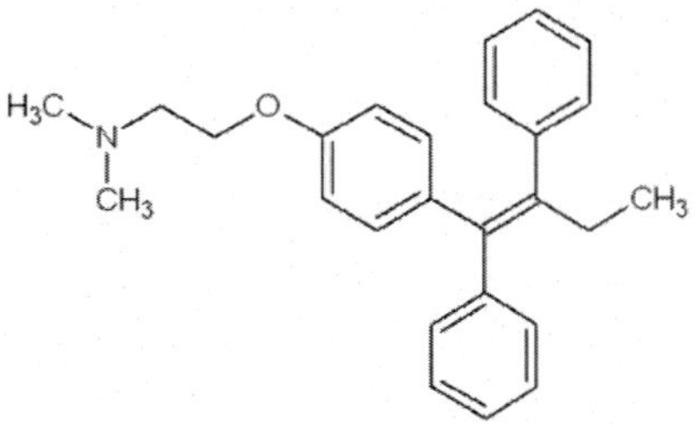

Tamoxifen

Figure 5. The selective estrogen receptor modulators Raloxifene and Tamoxifen.

Despite the beneficial effects of estrogen and/or HRT on inflammatory and immune responses after traumatic injury, there is a heavy body of evidence suggesting that hormone replacement has detrimental effects on multiple organ systems. These effects include the increased incidence of breast cancer and thromboembolic disease (Anderson et al. 2004; Cushman 2003; Grady et al. 2000; Manson et al. 2003; Störk et al. 2004). While consequences seem to be reduced with the use of low levels of estrogen, as with all therapeutic interventions, the benefits and risks need to be assessed on an individual basis, and also the topical treatment with estrogens should be administered with all necessary precautions, with careful monitoring of the areas of concentration and application, to prevent systemic side effects and minimizing interference with the physiology of the skin. Anyway, especially in relation to wound healing, it should be possible to directly target specific sites via the use of therapeutic agents whose biological action is localized around the area of administration. One way to achieve this effect is by a specifically designed soft drug (Bodor 1982; Bodor and Buchwald 2000, 2004). Soft drugs are pharmacologically active molecules as such, designed to undergo an expected and controllable metabolic deactivation after accomplishing their desired therapeutic effect. They have a molecular structure similar to a drug with a known activity and a specific metabolically sensitive moiety built into their structure to allow for a simple deactivation and detoxification after the desired therapeutic effect has been fulfilled. This strategy was used to synthesize a series of analogues of E2 derivatives containing metabolically unstable esters in strategic position (Figure 4). Among the E2 derivatives synthesized some compounds display a significant regenerative and anti-inflammatory activity, decrease the production of inflammatory molecules comparable to that of E2, and lack systemic effects when administered in the wound area of OVX mice (Brufani et al. 2009, 2017).

Another possible strategy to exploit the beneficial effects of estrogen lessening undesired side effects in target tissues, involves the use of selective estrogen receptor modulators (SERM), that are competitive partial agonists of the ER, producing estrogenic or antiestrogenic effects depending on the specific tissue and the percentage of intrinsic activity (Jordan et al. 2014). Raloxifene and tamoxifen (Figure 5) are most studied SERMs and have been proven effective in improving wound healing in OVX mice compared to estradiol (Hardman et al. 2008).

BIOLOGIC ESTROGENIC PRODUCTS

Natural products are traditionally the primary source of biologically active substances that is sieved for the discovery of lead compounds. Also in the case of biological wound healing products it is the estrogenic activity that is responsible for the acceleration of healing by increasing or modulating the inflammation mediators. Specifically, much attention has been focused on some phytoestrogens, particularly isoflavones, which have tissue-specific estrogen actions that can split the benefical biological effects from the undesired ones (Moraes et al. 2009; Accorsi-Neto et al. 2009).

Genistein (Figure 6) is considered a natural SERM with documented binding selectivity for the ER-β (Kuiper et al. 1998), but with binding affinity an order of magnitude lower than E2 (Pfitscher, Reiter, and Jungbauer 2008). Systemic chronic treatment of OVX rats with genistein hamper delayed wound healing, improving extracellular matrix remodeling and turnover. E2, raloxifene and genistein all significantly increase the wound healing and re-epithelialization, but the lowest genistein dose exerted a greater effect than the other treatments (Marini et al. 2010; Emmerson et al. 2010). Another study shows that genistein administration significantly accelerated the delayed wound healing in diabetic mice by improving angiogenesis. However, it seems that the effects of genistein on diabetic wound healing were only partially mediated by estrogen receptors (Tie et al. 2013).

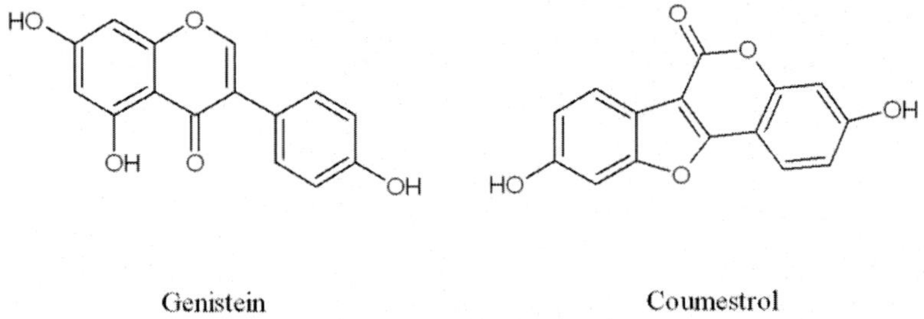

Genistein   Coumestrol

Figure 6. The phytoestrogens genistein and coumestrol.

Coumestrol (Figure 6) is a biologically active compound found in various species of the *Fabaceae* family, such as *Glycine max* and *Medicago sativa*. Some pharmacological activities have been ascribed to coumestrol, such as anti-inflammatory, anti-herpes HSV-1, and estrogen-like properties (Argenta et al. 2018; Chandsawangbhuwana and Baker 2014; You et al. 2017). It has been reported that coumestrol binds to the estrogen receptors ERα and ERβ, even at low concentrations, and for this reason, it was cataloged as a phytoestrogen (Al-Maharik and Botting 2004; Lorand, Vigh, and Garai 2010; Oseni et al. 2008). Coumestrol associated with hydroxypropyl-β-cyclodextrin (COU/HPβCD) was tested *in vitro* using a human gingival fibroblasts cell line and *in vivo* on male Wistar rats. The results indicated that the treatment carried out with COU/HPβCD showed high efficacy in wound healing with 50% wound healing achieved in a shorter period compared to the positive control (Bianchi et al. 2018).

REFERENCES

Abrahám, István M., Seong-Kyu Han, Martin G. Todman, Kenneth S. Korach, and Allan E. Herbison. 2003. "Estrogen Receptor β Mediates Rapid Estrogen Actions on Gonadotropin-Releasing Hormone Neurons *in Vivo.*" *J Neurosci* 23 (13): 5771–77. https://doi.org/10.1523/JNEUROSCI.23-13-05771.2003.

Accorsi-Neto, Alfeu, Mauro Haidar, Ricardo Simões, Manuel Simões, José Soares-Jr, and Edmund C. Baracat. 2009. "Effects of Isoflavones on the Skin of Postmenopausal Women: A Pilot Study." *Clinics* 64 (6): 505–10. https://doi.org/10.1590/S1807-59322009000600004.

Al-Maharik, Nawaf, and Nigel P Botting. 2004. "A New Short Synthesis of Coumestrol and Its Application for the Synthesis of [6,6a,11a-13C3]Coumestrol." *Tetrahedron* 60 (7): 1637–42. https://doi.org/10.1016/j.tet.2003.11.089.

Alexander, Stephen P. H., Alistair Mathie, and John A. Peters. 2011. "Guide to Receptors and Channels (GRAC), 5th Edition." *Brit J Pharmacol* 164: S1–324. https://doi.org/10.1111/j.1476-5381.2011.01649_1.x.

Anderson, G. L., M. Limacher, A. R. Assaf, T. Bassford, S. A. Beresford, H. Black, D. Bonds, et al. 2004. "Effects of Conjugated Equine Estrogen in Postmenopausal Women with Hysterectomy: The Women's Health Initiative Randomized Controlled Trial." *JAMA* 291 (14): 1701–12. https://doi.org/doi:10.1001/jama.291.14.1701.

Argenta, Débora Fretes, Juliana Bidone, Letícia Scherer Koester, Valquíria Link Bassani, Cláudia Maria Oliveira Simões, and Helder Ferreira Teixeira. 2018. "Topical Delivery of Coumestrol from Lipid

Nanoemulsions Thickened with Hydroxyethylcellulose for Antiherpes Treatment." *AAPS PharmSciTech* 19 (1): 192–200. https://doi.org/10. 1208/s12249-017-0828-8.

Ashcroft, Gillian S., Joanne Dodsworth, Egon van Boxtel, Roy W. Tarnuzzer, Michael A. Horan, Gregory S. Schultz, and Mark W. J. Ferguson. 1997. "Estrogen Accelerates Cutaneous Wound Healing Associated with an Increase of TGF1β Levels." *Nat Med* 3 (11): 1209–15. https://doi.org/10.1038/nm1197-1209.

Ashcroft, Gillian S., Teresa Greenwell-Wild, Michael A. Horan, Sharon M. Wahl, and Mark W. J. Ferguson. 1999. "Topical Estrogen Accelerates Cutaneous Wound Healing in Aged Humans Associated with an Altered Inflammatory Response." *Am J Pathol* 155 (4): 1137–46. https://doi.org/10.1016/S0002-9440(10)65217-0.

Ashcroft, Gillian S., and Stuart J. Mills. 2002. "Androgen Receptor-Mediated Inhibition of Cutaneous Wound Healing." *J Clin Invest* 110 (5): 615–24. https://doi.org/10.1172/JCI0215704.

Ashcroft, Gillian S., Stuart J. Mills, Ke Jian Lei, Linda Gibbons, Moon Jin Jeong, Marisu Taniguchi, Matthew Burow, Michael A. Horan, Sharon M. Wahl, and Toshinori Nakayama. 2003. "Estrogen Modulates Cutaneous Wound Healing by Downregulating Macrophage Migration Inhibitory Factor." *J Clin Invest* 111 (9): 1309–18. https://doi.org/10. 1172/JCI16288.

Ashworth, Jason J., J. V. Smyth, N. Pendleton, Michael A. Horan, A. Payton, J. Worthington, W. E. Ollier, and Gillian S. Ashcroft. 2008. "Polymorphisms Spanning the 0N Exon and Promoter of the Estrogen Receptor-Beta (ERβ) Gene ESR2 Are Associated with Venous Ulceration." *Clin Genet* 73 (1): 55–61. https://doi.org/10.1111/j.1399-0004.2007.00927.x.

Ashworth, Jason J., J. Vincent Smyth, Neil Pendleton, Michael Horan, Antony Payton, Jane Worthington, William E. Ollier, and Gillian S. Ashcroft. 2005. "The Dinucleotide (CA) Repeat Polymorphism of Estrogen Receptor Beta but Not the Dinucleotide (TA) Repeat Polymorphism of Estrogen Receptor Alpha Is Associated with Venous

Ulceration." *J Steroid Biochem* 97 (3): 266–70. https://doi.org/10.1016/j.jsbmb.2005.05.012.

Bai, Zhenlin, and Ronald Gust. 2009. "Breast Cancer, Estrogen Receptor and Ligands." *Arch Pharm* 342 (3): 133–49. https://doi.org/10.1002/ardp.200800174.

Bao, Philip, Arber Kodra, Marjana Tomic-Canic, Michael S. Golinko, H. Paul Ehrlich, and Harold Brem. 2009. "The Role of Vascular Endothelial Growth Factor in Wound Healing." *J Surg Res* https://doi.org/10.1016/j.jss.2008.04.023.

Barrientos, Stephan, Olivera Stojadinovic, Michael S. Golinko, Harold Brem, and Marjana Tomic-Canic. 2008. "Growth Factors and Cytokines in Wound Healing." *Wound Repair Regen* 16 (5): 585–601. https://doi.org/10.1111/j.1524-475x.2008.00410.x.

Bianchi, Sara E., Barbara E. K. Machado, Marília G. C. da Silva, Michelle M. A. da Silva, Lidiane Dal Bosco, Magno S. Marques, Ana P. Horn, et al. 2018. "Coumestrol/Hydroxypropyl-β-Cyclodextrin Association Incorporated in Hydroxypropyl Methylcellulose Hydrogel Exhibits Wound Healing Effect: *In Vitro* and *in Vivo* Study." *Eur J Pharm Sci* 119 (July): 179–88. https://doi.org/10.1016/j.ejps.2018.04.019.

Bochner, Bruce S., Ernest N. Charlesworth, Lawrence M. Lichtenstein, Claudia P. Derse, Steven Gillis, Charles A. Dinarello, and Robert P. Schleimer. 1990. "Interleukin-1 Is Released at Sites of Human Cutaneous Allergic Reactions." *J Allergy Clin Immunol* 86 (6 PART 1): 830–39. https://doi.org/10.1016/S0091-6749(05)80143-5.

Bodor, Nicholas. 1982. "Designing Safer Drug Based on the Soft Drug Approach." *Trends Pharmacol Sci* 3: 53–56.

Bodor, Nicholas, and Peter Buchwald. 2000. "Soft Drug Design: General Principles and Recent Applications." *Med Res Rev* 20 (1): 58–101. https://doi.org/10.1002/(SICI)1098-1128(200001)20:1<58::AID-MED3>3.0.CO;2-X.

Bodor, Nicholas, and Peter Buchwald. 2004. "Designing Safer (Soft) Drugs by Avoiding the Formation of Toxic and Oxidative Metabolites." *Mol Biotechnol* 26 (2): 123–32. https://doi.org/doi.org/10.1385/MB:26:2:123.

Brufani Mario, Francesca Ceccacci, Luigi Filocamo, Barbara Garofalo, Roberta Joudioux, Angela La Bella, Francesca Leonelli, et al. 2009. "Novel Locally Active Estrogens Accelerate Cutaneous Wound Healing. A Preliminary Study." *Mol Pharmaceutics* 6 (2): 543–56. https://doi.org/10.1021/mp800206b.

Brufani, Mario, Nicoletta Rizzi, Clara Meda, Luigi Filocamo, Francesca Ceccacci, Virginia D'Aiuto, Gabriele Bartoli, et al. 2017. "Novel Locally Active Estrogens Accelerate Cutaneous Wound Healing-Part 2." *Sci Rep* 7 (1): 2510. https://doi.org/10.1038/s41598-017-02820-y.

Buckley, Christopher D., Darrell Pilling, Janet M. Lord, Arne N. Akbar, Dagmar Scheel-Toellner, and Mike Salmon. 2001. "Fibroblasts Regulate the Switch from Acute Resolving to Chronic Persistent Inflammation." *Trends Immunol* 22 (4): 199–204. https://doi.org/10.1016/S1471-4906(01)01863-4.

Burger, Henry G. 2002. "Androgen Production in Women." *Fertil Steril* 77 (4): 4–6. https://doi.org/10.1016/S0015-0282(02)02985-0.

Chambliss, Ken L., Qian Wu, Sarah Oltmann, Eddy S. Konaniah, Michihisa Umetani, Kenneth S. Korach, Gail D. Thomas, et al. 2010. "Non-Nuclear Estrogen Receptor α Signaling Promotes Cardiovascular Protection but Not Uterine or Breast Cancer Growth in Mice." *J Clin Invest* 120 (7): 2319–30. https://doi.org/10.1172/JCI38291.

Chambliss, Ken L., Ivan S. Yuhanna, Richard G. W. Anderson, Michael E. Mendelsohn, and Philip W. Shaul. 2002. "ERβ Has Nongenomic Action in Caveolae." *Mol Endocrinol* 16 (5): 938–46. https://doi.org/10.1210/mend.16.5.0827.

Chandsawangbhuwana, Charlie, and Michael E. Baker. 2014. "3D Models of Human ERα and ERβ Complexed with Coumestrol." *Steroids* 80 (February): 37–43. https://doi.org/10.1016/j.steroids.2013.11.019.

Chen, Zhong, Ivan S. Yuhanna, Zoya Galcheva-Gargova, Richard H. Karas, Michael E. Mendelsohn, and Philip W. Shaul. 1999. "Estrogen Receptor α Mediates the Nongenomic Activation of Endothelial Nitric Oxide Synthase by Estrogen." *J Clin Invest* 103 (3): 401–6. https://doi.org/10.1172/JCI5347.

Corsini, Emanuela, Angelo Primavera, Marina Marinovich, and Corrado L. Galli. 1998. "Selective Induction of Cell-Associated Interleukin-1α in Murine Keratinocytes by Chemical Allergens." *Toxicology* 129 (2–3): 193–200. https://doi.org/10.1016/S0300-483X(98)00088-2.

Cushman, Mary. 2003. "Hormone Therapies and Vascular Outcomes: Who Is at Risk?" *J Thromb Thrombolys* 16 (1–2): 87–90. https://doi.org/10.1023/B:THRO.0000014601.57424.b8.

Diegelmann, Robert F., and Melissa C. Evans. 2004. "Wound Healing: An Overview of Acute, Fibrotic and Delayed Healing." *Front Biosci* 9 (January): 283–89. http://www.ncbi.nlm.nih.gov/pubmed/14766366.

Emmerson, Elaine, Laura Campbell, Gillian S. Ashcroft, and Matthew J. Hardman. 2010. "The Phytoestrogen Genistein Promotes Wound Healing by Multiple Independent Mechanisms." *Mol Cell Endocrinol* 321 (2): 184–93. https://doi.org/10.1016/j.mce.2010.02.026.

Evans, Rachel Anna, Ya Chung Tian, Robert Steadman, and Aled Owain Phillips. 2003. "TGF-B1-Mediated Fibroblast-Myofibroblast Terminal Differentiation - The Role of Smad Proteins." *Exp Cell Res* 282 (2): 90–100. https://doi.org/10.1016/S0014-4827(02)00015-0.

Figtree, Gemma A., Denise McDonald, Hugh Watkins, and Keith M. Channon. 2003. "Truncated Estrogen Receptor α 46-KDa Isoform in Human Endothelial Cells." *Circulation* 107 (1): 120–26. https://doi.org/10.1161/01.cir.0000043805.11780.f5.

Filardo, Edward J., Jeffrey A. Quinn, Kirby I. Bland, and A. Raymond Frackelton. 2000. "Estrogen-Induced Activation of Erk-1 and Erk-2 Requires the G Protein-Coupled Receptor Homolog, GPR30, and Occurs via Trans-Activation of the Epidermal Growth Factor Receptor through Release of HB-EGF." *Mol Endocrinol* 14 (10): 1649–60. https://doi.org/10.1210/mend.14.10.0532.

Filardo, Edward J., and Peter Thomas. 2012. "Minireview: G Protein-Coupled Estrogen Receptor-1, GPER-1: Its Mechanism of Action and Role in Female Reproductive Cancer, Renal and Vascular Physiology." *Endocrinology* 153 (7): 2953–62. https://doi.org/10.1210/en.2012-1061.

Freedberg, Irwin M., Marjana Tomic-Canic, Mayumi Komine, and Miroslav Blumenberg. 2001. "Keratins and the Keratinocyte Activation Cycle." *J Invest Dermatol* 116 (5): 633–40. https://doi.org/ 10.1046/j.0022-202x.2001.doc.x.

Gabbiani, G., B. J. Hirschel, G. B. Ryan, P. R. Statkov, and G. Majno. 1972. "Granulation Tissue as a Contractile Organ. A Study of Structure and Function." *J Exp Med* 135 (4): 719–34. https://doi.org/ 10.1084/jem.135.4.719.

Gilliver, Stephen C., Jason J. Ashworth, Stuart J. Mills, Matthew J. Hardman, and Gillian S. Ashcroft. 2006. "Androgens Modulate the Inflammatory Response during Acute Wound Healing." *J Cell Sci* 119 (4): 722–32. https://doi.org/10.1242/jcs.02786.

Gilliver, Stephen C., Elaine Emmerson, Jürgen Bernhagen, and Matthew J. Hardman. 2011. "MIF: A Key Player in Cutaneous Biology and Wound Healing." *Exp Dermatol* 20 (1): 1–6. https://doi.org/10.1111/ j.1600-0625.2010.01194.x.

Gilliver, Stephen C., Jayalath P. D. Ruckshanthi, Matthew J. Hardman, Toshinori Nakayama, and Gillian S. Ashcroft. 2008. "Sex Dimorphism in Wound Healing: The Roles of Sex Steroids and Macrophage Migration Inhibitory Factor." *Endocrinology* 149 (11): 5747–57. https://doi.org/10.1210/en.2008-0355.

Gilliver, Stephen C., Jayalath P. D. Ruckshanthi, Matthew J. Hardman, L. A.H. Zeef, and Gillian S. Ashcroft. 2009. "5α-Dihydrotestosterone (DHT) Retards Wound Closure by Inhibiting Re-Epithelialization." *J Pathol* 217 (1): 73–82. https://doi.org/10.1002/path.2444.

Gilliver, Stephen C., Fred Wu, and Gillian S. Ashcroft. 2003. "Regulatory Roles of Androgens in Cutaneous Wound Healing." *Thromb Haemostasis* 90 (6): 978–85. https://doi.org/10.1160/TH03-05-0302.

Glaros, Trevor, Michelle Larsen, and Liwu Li. 2009. "Macrophages and Fibroblasts during Inflammation, Tissue Damage and Organ Injury." *Front Biosci* Volume (14): 3988. https://doi.org/10.2741/3506.

Grady, Deborah, Nanette K Wenger, David Herrington, Steven Khan, Curt Furberg, Donald Hunninghake, Erie Vittinghoff, and Stephen Hulley. 2000. "Postmenopausal Hormone Therapy Increases Risk for Venous

Thromboembolic Disease The Heart and Estrogen/Progestin Replacement Study." *Ann Intern Med* 132 (9): 689–96. https://doi.org/10.7326/0003-4819-132-9-200005020-00002.

Gulshan, S., A. B. McCruden, and W. H. Stimson. 1990. "Oestrogen Receptors in Macrophages." *Scand J Immunol* 31 (6): 691–97. https://doi.org/10.1111/j.1365-3083.1990.tb02820.x.

Gurtner, Geoffrey C., Sabine Werner, Yann Barrandon, and Michael T. Longaker. 2008. "Wound Repair and Regeneration." *Nature* 453: 314–21. https://doi.org/10.1038/nature07039.

Hackam, David J., and Henri R. Ford. 2002. "Cellular, Biochemical, and Clinical Aspects of Wound Healing." *Surg Infect* 3 (s1): s23–35. https://doi.org/10.1089/sur.2002.3.s1-23.

Hamilton, Katherine J., Sylvia C. Hewitt, Yukitomo Arao, and Kenneth S. Korach. 2017. "Estrogen Hormone Biology." *Curr Top Dev Biol* 125: 109–46. https://doi.org/10.1002/cncr.27633.

Hantash, Basil M., Longmei Zhao, Joseph A. Knowles, and Peter H. Lorenz. 2008. "Adult and Fetal Wound Healing." *Front Biosci* 13: 51–61. http://www.ahrq.gov/clinic/epcsums/woundsum.htm.

Harding, Keith G., Keith Moore, and Tania J. Phillips. 2005. "Wound Chronicity and Fibroblast Senescence - Implications for Treatment." *Intm Wound J* 2 (4). https://doi.org/10.1111/j.1742-4801.2005.00149.x.

Hardman, Matthew J., Elaine Emmerson, Laura Campbell, and Gillian S. Ashcroft. 2008. "Selective Estrogen Receptor Modulators Accelerate Cutaneous Wound Healing in Ovariectomized Female Mice." *Endocrinology* 149 (2): 551–57. https://doi.org/10.1210/en.2007-1042.

Hardman, Matthew J., Alexander Waite, Leo Zeef, Matthew Burow, Toshinori Nakayama, and Gillian S. Ashcroft. 2005. "Macrophage Migration Inhibitory Factor: A Central Regulator of Wound Healing." *Am J Pathol* 167 (6): 1561–74. https://doi.org/10.1016/S0002-9440(10)61241-2.

Hewitt, Sylvia C., and Kenneth S. Korach. 2018. "Estrogen Receptors: New Directions in the New Millennium." *Endocrinol Rev* 39 (5): 664–75. https://doi.org/10.1210/er.2018-00087.

Hinz, Boris, Sem H. Phan, Victor J. Thannickal, Marco Prunotto, Alexis Desmoulire, John Varga, Olivier De Wever, Marc Mareel, and Giulio Gabbiani. 2012. "Recent Developments in Myofibroblast Biology: Paradigms for Connective Tissue Remodeling." *Am J Pathol* 180 (4): 1340–55. https://doi.org/10.1016/j.ajpath.2012.02.004.

Hynes, Richard O. 2009. "Extracellular Matrix: Not Just Pretty Fibrils." *Science* 326 (5957): 1216–1219. https://doi.org/10.1126/science.117 6009.

Jordan, V. Craig, Russell McDaniel, Fadeke Agboke, and Philipp Y. Maximov. 2014. "The Evolution of Nonsteroidal Antiestrogens to Become Selective Estrogen Receptor Modulators." *Steroids* 90: 3–12. https://doi.org/10.1039/b800799c.O.

Kanda, Naoko, and Shinichi Watanabe. 2004a. "17β-Estradiol Stimulates the Growth of Human Keratinocytes by Inducing Cyclin D2 Expression." *J Invest Dermatol* 123 (2): 319–28. https://doi.org/10.1111/j.0022-202X.2004.12645.x.

Kanda, Naoko, and Shinichi Watanabe. 2004b. "17β-Estradiol the Production of Granulocyte-Macrophage Colony-Stimulating Factor in Human Keratinocytes." *J Invest Dermatol* 123 (2): 329–37. https://doi.org/10.1111/j.0022-202X.2004.23231.x.

Kang, Lianguo, Xintian Zhang, Yan Xie, Yaping Tu, Dong Wang, Zhenming Liu, and Zhao-Yi Wang. 2010. "Involvement of Estrogen Receptor Variant ER-A36, Not GPR30, in Nongenomic Estrogen Signaling." *Mol Endocrinol* 24 (4): 709–21. https://doi.org/10.1210/me.2009-0317.

Kirsner, Robert S., and William H. Eaglstein. 1993. "The Wound Healing Process." *Dermatol Clin* 11 (4): 629–40. https://doi.org/10.1016/S0733-8635(18)30216-X.

Kondo, Toshikazu, and Yuko Ishida. 2010. "Molecular Pathology of Wound Healing." *Forensic Sci Int* 203 (1–3): 93–98. https://doi.org/10.1016/j.forsciint.2010.07.004.

Kuiper, George G. J. M., Josephine G. Lemmen, B. O. Carlsson, J. Christopher Corton, Stephen H. Safe, Paul T. Van Der Saag, Bart Van Der Burg, and Jan-Åke Gustafsson. 1998. "Interaction of Estrogenic

Chemicals and Phytoestrogens with Estrogen Receptor." *Endocrinology* 139 (10): 4252–63. https://doi.org/10.1210/endo.139. 10.6216.

Kumar, Raj, Mikhail N. Zakharov, Shagufta H. Khan, Rika Miki, Hyeran Jang, Gianluca Toraldo, Rajan Singh, Shalender Bhasin, and Ravi Jasuja. 2011. "The Dynamic Structure of the Estrogen Receptor." *J Amino Acids* 2011: 1–7. https://doi.org/10.4061/2011/812540.

Lawrence, Thomas W. 1998. "Physiology of the Acute Wound." *Clin Plast Surg* 25 (3): 321–40. https://www.ncbi.nlm.nih.gov/pubmed/9696896.

Leng, Lin, Christine N. Metz, Yan Fang, Jing Xu, Seamas Donnelly, John Baugh, Thomas Delohery, Yibang Chen, Robert A. Mitchell, and Richard Bucala. 2003. "MIF Signal Transduction Initiated by Binding to CD74." *J Exp Med* 197 (11): 1467–76. https://doi.org/10.1084/jem.20030286.

Li, L., M. P. Haynes, and J. R. Bender. 2003. "Plasma Membrane Localization and Function of the Estrogen Receptor Alpha Variant (ER46) in Human Endothelial Cells." *Proc Natl Acad Sci USA* 100 (8): 4807–12. https://doi.org/10.1073/pnas.0831079100.

Lombardi, G., S. Zarrilli, A. Colao, L. Paesano, C. Di Somma, F. Rossi, and M. De Rosa. 2001. "Estrogens and Health in Males." *Mol Cell Endocrinol* 178 (1–2): 51–55. https://doi.org/10.1016/S0303-7207(01)00420-8.

Lorand, T., E. Vigh, and J. Garai. 2010. "Hormonal Action of Plant Derived and Anthropogenic Non-Steroidal Estrogenic Compounds: Phytoestrogens and Xenoestrogens." *Curr Med Chem* 17 (30): 3542–74. https://doi.org/10.2174/092986710792927813.

Maggiolini, Marcello, Adele Vivacqua, Giovanna Fasanella, Anna Grazia Recchia, Diego Sisci, Vincenzo Pezzi, Daniela Montanaro, Anna Maria Musti, Didier Picard, and Sebastiano Andò. 2004. "The G Protein-Coupled Receptor GPR30 Mediates c-Fos up-Regulation by 17β-Estradiol and Phytoestrogens in Breast Cancer Cells." *J Biol Chem* 279 (26): 27008–16. https://doi.org/10.1074/jbc.M403588200.

Manavathi, Bramanandam, and Rakesh Kumar. 2006. "Steering Estrogen Signals from the Plasma Membrane to the Nucleus: Two Sides of the

Coin." *J Cell Physiol* 207 (3): 594–604. https://doi.org/10.1002/jcp. 20551.

Manson, JoAnn E., Judith Hsia, Karen C. Johnson, Jacques E. Rossouw, Annlouise R. Assaf, Norman L. Lasser, Maurizio Trevisan, et al. 2003. "Estrogen plus Progestin and the Risk of Coronary Heart Disease." *New Engl J Med* 349 (6): 523–34. https://doi.org/10.1056/NEJ Moa030808.

Marini, H., F. Polito, D. Altavilla, N. Irrera, L. Minutoli, M. Calò, Eb Adamo, M. Vaccaro, F. Squadrito, and A. Bitto. 2010. "Genistein Aglycone Improves Skin Repair in an Incisional Model of Wound Healing: A Comparison with Raloxifene and Oestradiol in Ovariectomized Rats." *Brit J Pharmacol* 160 (5): 1185–94. https://doi.org/10.1111/j.1476-5381.2010.00758.x.

Mills, Stuart J., Jason J. Ashworth, Stephen C. Gilliver, Matthew J. Hardman, and Gillian S. Ashcroft. 2005. "The Sex Steroid Precursor DHEA Accelerates Cutaneous Wound Healing Via the Estrogen Receptors." *J Invest Dermatol* 125 (5): 1053–62. https://doi.org/10. 1111/j.0022-202X.2005.23926.x.

Monaco, JoAn L, and W Thomas Lawrence. 2003. "Acute Wound Healing an Overview." *Clin Plast Surg* 30 (1): 1–12. http://www.ncbi.nlm.nih. gov/pubmed/12636211.

Moraes, Andrea B., Mauro A. Haidar, José Maria Soares, Manuel J. Simões, Edmund C. Baracat, and Marisa T. Patriarca. 2009. "The Effects of Topical Isoflavones on Postmenopausal Skin: Double-Blind and Randomized Clinical Trial of Efficacy." *Eur J Obstet Gyn R B* 146 (2): 188–92. https://doi.org/10.1016/j.ejogrb.2009.04.007.

Moro, Laura, Stefania Reineri, Daniela Piranda, Daniela Pietrapiana, Paolo Lova, Alessandra Bertoni, Andrea Graziani, et al. 2005. "Nongenomic Effects of 17β-Estradiol in Human Platelets: Potentiation of Thrombin-Induced Aggregation through Estrogen Receptor β and Src Kinase." *Blood* 105 (1): 115–21. https://doi.org/10.1182/blood-2003-11-3840.

Mukai, Kanae, Tamae Urai, Kimi Asano, Yukari Nakajima, and Toshio Nakatani. 2016a. "Evaluation of Effects of Topical Estradiol Benzoate Application on Cutaneous Wound Healing in Ovariectomized Female

Mice." *PLoS ONE* 11 (9): 1–15. https://doi.org/10.1371/journal. pone.0163560.

Mukai, Kanae, Yukari Nakajima, Tamae Urai, Emi Komatsu, Nasruddin, Junko Sugama, and Toshio Nakatani. 2016b. "17□-Estradiol Administration Promotes Delayed Cutaneous Wound Healing in 40-Week Ovariectomised Female Mice." *Int Wound J* 13 (5): 636–44. https://doi.org/10.1111/iwj.12336.

Murphy, Jo Ellen, Caroline Robert, and Thomas S. Kupper. 2000. "Interleukin-1 and Cutaneous Inflammation: A Crucial Link between Innate and Acquired Immunity." *J Invest Dermatol* 114 (3): 602–8. https://doi.org/10.1046/j.1523-1747.2000.00917.x.

Nakajima, Yukari, Yuka Eno, Mariko Hirata, Sawako Kobori, Ayano Sugiura, Maiko Takeuchi, Miho Taniguchi, et al. 2013. "Is Estrogen Effective for Full-Thickness Cutaneous Wound Healing in Young Male Mice?" *Wounds* 25 (10): 278–86. http://www.woundsresearch. com/article/estrogen-effective-full-thickness-cutaneous-wound-healing-young-male-mice.

Nurden, Alan T., Paquita Nurden, Mikel Sanchez, Isabel Andia, and Eduardo Anitua. 2008. "Platelets and Wound Healing." *Front Biosci* 13 (May): 3532–48. http://www.ncbi.nlm.nih.gov/pubmed/18508453.

Oseni, Tawakalitu, Roshani Patel, Jennifer Pyle, V Craig Jordan, Craig Jordan, and Alfred G Knudson Chair. 2008. "Selective Estrogen Receptor Modulators and Phytoestrogens." *Planta Med* 74: 1656–65. https://doi.org/10.1055/s-0028-1088304.

Pelletier, G., and L. Ren. 2004. "Localization of Sex Steroid Receptors in Human Skin." *Histol Histopathol* 19 (2): 629–36. https://doi.org/10. 14670/HH-19.629.

Pfitscher, Angelika, Evelyne Reiter, and Alois Jungbauer. 2008. "Receptor Binding and Transactivation Activities of Red Clover Isoflavones and Their Metabolites." *J Steroid Biochem* 112 (1–3): 87–94. https://doi. org/10.1016/j.jsbmb.2008.08.007.

Prossnitz, Eric R., Jeffrey B. Arterburn, Harriet O. Smith, Tudor I. Oprea, Larry A. Sklar, and Helen J. Hathaway. 2008. "Estrogen Signaling through the Transmembrane G Protein–Coupled Receptor GPR30."

Ann Rev Physiol 70 (1): 165–90. https://doi.org/10.1146/annurev. physiol.70.113006.100518.

Razandi, Mahnaz, Ali Pedram, Istvan Merchenthaler, Geoffrey L. Greene, and Ellis R. Levin. 2004. "Plasma Membrane Estrogen Receptors Exist and Functions as Dimers." *Mol Endocrinol* 18 (12): 2854–65. https://doi.org/10.1210/me.2004-0115.

Revankar, Chetana M., Daniel F. Cimino, Larry A. Sklar, Jeffrey B. Arterburn, and Eric R. Prossnitz. 2005. "A Transmembrane Intracellular Estrogen Receptor Mediates Rapid Cell Signaling." *Science* 307 (5715): 1625–30. https://doi.org/10.1126/science. 1106943.

Schultz, Gregory S., and Annette Wysocki. 2009. "Interactions between Extracellular Matrix and Growth Factors in Wound Healing." *Wound Repair Regen* 17 (2): 153–62. https://doi.org/10.1111/j.1524-475X. 2009.00466.x.

Serini, Guido, Marie-Luce Bochaton-Piallat, Patricia Ropraz, Antoine Geinoz, Laura Borsi, Luciano Zardi, and Giulio Gabbiani. 1998. "The Fibronectin Domain ED-A Is Crucial for Myofibroblastic Phenotype Induction by Transforming Growth Factor-1." *J Cell Biol* Vol. 142. http://www.jcb.org.

Singer, Adam J., and Richard A. F. Clark. 1999. "Cutaneous Wound Healing." *New Engl J Med* 341 (10): 738–46. https://doi.org/10.1056/ NEJM199909023411006.

Sjostedt, S. 1953. "The Effect of Diethylstilbenediol on the Healing of Wounds in the Human Vagina." *Acta Endocrinol* 12 (3): 260–63. http://www.ncbi.nlm.nih.gov/pubmed/13050301.

Sjövall, Alf. 1947. "The Influence of Oestrogen upon the Healing of Vaginal Wounds in Rats." *Acta Obstet Gyn Scan* 27 (1): 1–10. https://doi.org/10.3109/00016344709159873.

Stevenson, Susan, and Julie Thornton. 2007. "Effect of Estrogens on Skin Aging and the Potential Role of SERMs Estrogens and Skin Biology." *Clin Inter Aging* 2 (3): 283–97. https://doi.org/doi.org/10.2147/ CIA.S798.

Störk, Stefan, Yvonne T. Van Der Schouw, Diederick E. Grobbee, and Michiel L. Bots. 2004. "Estrogen, Inflammation and Cardiovascular Risk in Women: A Critical Appraisal." *Trends Endocrin Met* 15 (2): 66–72. https://doi.org/10.1016/j.tem.2004.01.005.

Tassi, Elena, Kevin McDonnell, Krissa A. Gibby, Jason U. Tilan, Sung E. Kim, David P. Kodack, Marcel O. Schmidt, et al. 2011. "Impact of Fibroblast Growth Factor-Binding Protein1 Expression on Angiogenesis and Wound Healing." *Am J Pathol* 179 (5): 2220–32. https://doi.org/10.1016/j.ajpath.2011.07.043.

Thomas, Peter, Y. Pang, Edward J. Filardo, and J. Dong. 2005. "Identity of an Estrogen Membrane Receptor Coupled to a G Protein in Human Breast Cancer Cells." *Endocrinology* 146 (2): 624–32. https://doi.org/10.1210/en.2004-1064.

Thornton, M. J., A. H. Taylor, F. Al-Azzawi, C. C. Lyon, J. O'Driscoll, and A. G. Messenger. 2003. "Oestrogen Receptor Beta Is the Predominant Oestrogen Receptor in Human Scalp Skin Male or Female Skin. The Wide Distribution of ER in Human Skin." *Exp Dermatol* 12 (2): 181–90. https://doi.org/10.1034/j.1600-0625.2003.120209.x.

Tie, Lu, Yu An, Jing Han, Yuan Xiao, Yilixiati Xiaokaiti, Shengjun Fan, Shaoqiang Liu, Alex F. Chen, and Xuejun Li. 2013. "Genistein Accelerates Refractory Wound Healing by Suppressing Superoxide and FoxO1/iNOS Pathway in Type 1 Diabetes." *J Nutr Biochem* 24 (1): 88–96. https://doi.org/10.1016/j.jnutbio.2012.02.011.

Trenti, Annalisa, Serena Tedesco, Carlotta Boscaro, Lucia Trevisi, Chiara Bolego, and Andrea Cignarella. 2018. "Estrogen, Angiogenesis, Immunity and Cell Metabolism: Solving the Puzzle." *Int J Mol Sci* 19 (3): 859–74. https://doi.org/10.3390/ijms19030859.

Velnar, T., T. Bailey, and V. Smrkolj. 2009. "The Wound Healing Process: An Overview of the Cellular and Molecular Mechanisms." *J Int Med Res* Vol. 37.

Verdier-Sevrain, S., M. Yaar, J. Cantatore, A. Traish, and B. A. Gilchrest. 2004. "Estradiol Induces Proliferation of Keratinocytes via a Receptor

Mediated Mechanism." *FASEB J* 18 (11): 1252–54. https://doi.org/10.1096/fj.03-1088fje.

Wilkinson, Holly N., and Matthew J. Hardman. 2017. "The Role of Estrogen in Cutaneous Ageing and Repair." *Maturitas* 103: 60–64. https://doi.org/10.1016/j.maturitas.2017.06.026.

You, Jae-Seek, In-A Cho, Kyeong-Rok Kang, Ji-Su Oh, Sang-Joun Yu, Gyeong-Je Lee, Yo-Seob Seo, et al. 2017. "Coumestrol Counteracts Interleukin-1β-Induced Catabolic Effects by Suppressing Inflammation in Primary Rat Chondrocytes." *Inflammation* 40 (1): 79–91. https://doi.org/10.1007/s10753-016-0455-7.

In: A Closer Look at Wound Infections …   ISBN: 978-1-53616-816-7
Editor: Joseph E. Keel   © 2020 Nova Science Publishers, Inc.

Chapter 4

IMPACT OF PHOTOBIOMODULATION THERAPY ON CHRONIC WOUND HEALING

Nicolette Nadene Houreld* and Sandy Winfield Jere
Laser Research Centre, Faculty of Health Sciences,
University of Johannesburg, Johannesburg, South Africa

ABSTRACT

As a complex and highly regulated process occurring in overlapping phases, wound healing is key to retaining physiological function of the skin. Characterised by an excessive and unrelenting inflammatory phase, persistent infection, and diminished cellular response to environmental stimuli, chronic wounds significantly pose a burden to patients and service providers, including the entire healthcare system. Chronic wounds include venous, ischemic and diabetic foot ulcers, and purulent wounds, such as surgical site infections. Most distressing, the response of chronic wounds to exorbitantly expensive conventional therapeutic methods is often diminished, and once healed these wounds are frequently considered "high risk for recurrence", particularly in the case of diabetic foot ulcers. With the projected epidemic of diabetes mellitus and an aging population in developing countries, it is important to substantiate cheaper

---

* Corresponding Author's E-mail: nhoureld@uj.ac.za.

and safer therapeutic techniques for the management of chronic wounds to allow health care providers access to treatment alternatives for their patients. For this reason, the development of innovative non-invasive therapeutic modalities is crucial. For some time now, photobiomodulation therapy (PBMT), formally referred to as low-level light/laser therapy (LLLT), has been used to induce physiological changes and therapeutic benefits. Despite the overwhelming evidence regarding its therapeutic capability, PBMT is not universally accepted as the induced effects at a tissue, cellular and molecular level are not completely understood, and mistrust or cynicism towards alternative and unconventional medicine. PBMT involves the use of low-powered (usually less than 1 W/cm^2) light emitting diodes (LEDs), lasers or broadband light, mostly in the visible red and near infrared (NIR) light spectrum (600 – 1,100 nm). It is used in a wide variety of applications, and is typically used to alleviate pain, reduce inflammation and oedema, and speed up healing or induce healing in non-responsive chronic wounds of a wide range of aetiologies. Further evidence of the efficiency of existing and future wound therapies is necessitated for their acceptance and appropriate use. This chapter explores the impact of PBMT on wound healing and the basic biochemical reactions involved.

Keywords: photobiomodulation, lasers, light emitting diodes, wound healing, chronic wounds

INTRODUCTION

Wound Healing

According to the World Health Organisation (WHO) the phrase "wound healing" comprises all types of wounds, burns, and ulcerations (World Health Organisation, 2010). The regeneration and repair processes that follows the onset of tissue injury, usually due to trauma or a pathological condition, involves a chain of cellular and molecular activities aiming at restoration of the injured tissue.

Wound healing is split into four overlapping phases, namely heamostasis which begins immediately after injury and involves formation of a clot to minimise blood loss and provide a matrix for infiltrating cells; inflammation which begins shortly after injury and is aimed at cleaning up cellular debris and preventing bacterial infection; proliferation which starts within days after injury and is concerned with the synthesis of new granulation tissue; and lastly tissue remodelling/maturation which begins 2 to 3 weeks after injury and is directed at converting granulation tissue into a mature scar, and typically lasts a year or longer. Wound healing occurs via a combination of complex and dynamic processes coordinated by soluble mediators released by both parenchymal and blood cells (Gonzalez et al. 2016). Cutaneous wounds heal by the resurfacing of epithelial cells followed by wound reduction, and is dependent on the features of the wound including the depth, location, size, bacterial contamination and patient health (Sorg et al. 2017). Under normal circumstances, the process of cutaneous wound healing is well organised, and leads to a predictable tissue restoration where different cells types, including keratinocytes and fibroblasts, play a significant role in the reestablishment of tissue integrity (Demidova-Rice et al. 2012).

The desired final consequence of the wound healing process is the formation of tissue structure with similar functional capability as intact skin. However, complete regeneration is exceptional to early foetal healing as cutaneous wound healing may result in moderately restored tissue, with physical and functional competence that is not identical to the original tissue. Alterations to healing processes extend both the damage and repair of tissue, and in pathobiologic situations leads to the development of non-healing or difficult to heal chronic wounds (Li et al. 2007). Atypical wound healing processes are rarely seen in normal, healthy individuals, and are frequently linked to age and underlying defects (Han and Ceilley, 2017). Assessment of underlying pathologies and contemplation for improved therapeutic agents should be taken into consideration when wounds fail to attain adequate healing after 4 weeks of standard care (Frykberg and Banks, 2015).

Chronic Wound Healing

Chronic wounds represent a major challenge and cost burden for global healthcare systems, and have distressing effects on patients and society at large. The burden of chronic wounds is underrated and increasing as a result of the growing elderly population and prevalence of chronic diseases, and frequently these wounds advance into critical complications including limb amputations and premature death (Järbrink et al. 2017). Studies elucidate that chronic wounds not only develop due to advanced age, but also the presence of comorbidities frequently observed among this population such as diabetes, neuropathy, vascular disease and nephropathy (Samaniego-Ruiz et al. 2018). Chronic wounds may be described as those that fail to progress through the normal and timely tissue restorative process within a specified timeframe, or those that proceed through the restorative process but do not establish a lasting tissue structure and functional outcome (Järbrink et al. 2017). The repair of chronic wounds has become a specialty in which health workers frequently use advanced therapies (costing 2% to 3% of healthcare resources in developed countries) including extracellular matrices (ECMs), negative pressure wound therapy (NPWT), growth factors and bioengineered skin (Frykberg and Banks, 2015). Based on the causative aetiology, chronic wounds are categorised into diabetic, pressure and vascular (arterial and venous) ulcers, and in developed countries it is estimated that 2% of the population suffer from a chronic wound at least once during their lifetime (Järbrink et al. 2017). On average, chronic lower limb ulcers last for 12 to 13 months, and recur in 60% to 70% of cases (Frykberg and Banks, 2015). This may lead to decreased mobility and productivity which in itself leads to further co-morbidity, and increased pain and discomfort, ultimately resulting in reduced quality of life.

The microenvironment in chronic wounds is fundamentally transformed with disrupted interaction of cytokines and growth factors, affecting the typical wound healing phases. These wounds typically get stuck in the inflammatory phase, and present with elevated proinflammatory cytokines, reactive oxygen species (ROS), senescent cells, matrix metalloproteinases (MMPs) and proteases that degrade and inhibit the deposition of new ECM and cell migration, and reduced growth factors, protease inhibitors, stem cells, ECM deposition and angiogenesis. Furthermore, MMPs significantly reduce growth factors and cytokines that are critical in the regulation of the wound microenvironment and wound healing progression (Turner and Badylak, 2015). There is also the high probability of persistent bacterial wound infection, despite an incessant inflammatory phase. There are reports that fibroblasts, keratinocytes, endothelial cells and macrophages from chronic wounds are senescent and have a reduced proliferative ability due to oxidative stress. This may have effects on the DNA damage related cell cycle arrest, and may result in reduced function of intracellular signal transduction pathways (Bitar, 2012). Qing (2017) expounded on the molecular effects in chronic wounds, including in diabetic ulcers, and indicated that the diminished production of cytokines/growth factors and their receptors, collagen and granulation tissue, reduced fibroblast proliferation and migration, and increased MMPs that break the functional characteristics of the epidermal barrier are all responsible for delayed and dysfunctional healing.

A thorough management of chronic wounds includes the reduction of factors that promote delayed healing. Reassessment of the underlying cause and consideration for innovative therapeutic methods should be undertaken once a wound fail to attain satisfactory healing following standard treatment methods (Frykberg and Banks, 2015). It is not surprising so far that the subject of wound healing in research is extremely active considering the impact that chronic wounds present worldwide on both patient care and economics. Furthermore, due to unsatisfactory efficacy of conventional treatment methodologies and development of antimicrobial resistant pathogens, new research on wound healing have focused on novel methods that may be seen as helpful in enhancing the healing process (Han and Ceilley, 2017). There is increasing evidence that the use of non-pharmacological/non-invasive restorative methods using light energy, also referred to as photobiomodulation (PBM), formally denoted as low level light/laser therapy (LLLT), could enhance wound healing (Jere et al. 2019), and its use could be advantageous over administered treatment methods that have the risk of both localised and systemic after effects.

Photobiomodulation Therapy

PBMT is a term used to describe a therapy which makes use of light at specific wavelengths and is based on the principles of photobiomodulation (PBM), which in itself is the mechanism of stimulating biological systems in organisms using light (photon energy). PBM relies on the absorption of non-ionising optical radiation or photons, typically in the visible (red) and near-infrared (NIR) spectrum, from lasers, light emitting diodes (LEDs) and broadband light (with filters). These photons are absorbed by endogenous chromophores (structures within tissue/cell which absorbs light) which results in photochemical and photophysical responses without generating huge amounts of heat and without inducing thermal tissue damage. PBMT has been in use by clinicians since the late 1960s and involves irradiating diseased/stressed/damaged tissue with relatively low-powered light devices, most commonly lasers or LED arrays. The absorbed photons speed-up and activate an array of cellular processes, leading to downstream physiological effects which engenders improved healing, decreased inflammation and oedema, and reduced pain. Generally, PBMT is performed with red and/or NIR light (600 – 1,100 nm) with an output power of $1 - 10,000$ mW and using a power density that does not induce tissue thermal damage (less than 1 W/cm^2, depending on the wavelength and tissue type). An energy density or fluence of $0.1 - 100$ J/cm^2 is usually applied (Hamblin et al. 2018). Wavelengths below 600 nm are typically not used in PBMT since chromophores found in the tissue, namely haemoglobin and melanin, have high absorption bands at these shorter wavelengths. Similarly, wavelengths above 1150 nm are not used since water absorbs at these higher wavelengths.

For more than 50 years since its discovery, PBMT has not gained a universal acceptance, largely due to incomplete clarity on the tissue, cellular and molecular processes it provides, lack of knowledge and consensus of treatment parameters to use, and distrust or cynicism of unconventional (alternative/complementary) medicine. The basic mechanism of PBM is centred on the theory of biostimulatory action that helps in modifying intracellular behaviour, resulting from the activation of either the mitochondrial respiratory chain or the calcium channels on the mitochondrial membrane causing cellular alterations (Kohale et al. 2018). Scientists have elucidated the involvement of cytochrome c oxidase (COX), mitochondrial unit IV (chromophore) of the respiratory chain. Exact reactions that trail this initial photon-absorption event of COX remains incompletely understood. What is known is that COX is able to absorb light in the visible red and NIR spectrum leading to an increased mitochondrial membrane potential, electron translocation and adenosine triphosphate (ATP) production (De Freitas and Hamblin, 2016; Houreld et al. 2012; Zungu et al. 2009). ATP is a central metabolite that provides cellular energy to drive many processes, it is also an important extracellular signalling molecule.

PBM photodissociates inhibitory nitric oxide (NO) from COX, where it is bound to the COX haeme and copper centres and thus allows for normal cellular respiration to occur/increase, this process leads to increased mitochondrial membrane potential, which in turn leads to increased intracellular ROS, ATP and cyclic adenosine monophosphate (cAMP), NO, calcium ions (Ca^{2+}) and initiation of factors for transcription (Hamblin, 2016). The photobiostimulatory effect largely promotes cell proliferation, differentiation, migration and survival, and literature supports that the effects of PBM are due to the increase in "good" ROS that has the ability to activate signalling pathways sensitive to cellular redox variations (De Freitas and Hamblin, 2016). It has also been noted that although PBM produces increased ROS in normal cells, ROS levels are decreased in oxidatively stressed cells (Hamblin et al. 2018). Downstream transcriptional factors, including nuclear factor kappa light chain enhancer of activated B cells (NF-kB), are initiated (Figure 1) leading to gene expression for various proteins responsible for cell proliferation, migration, collagen production, anti-apoptosis, neoangiogenesis and tissue restoration (Hamblin, 2010).

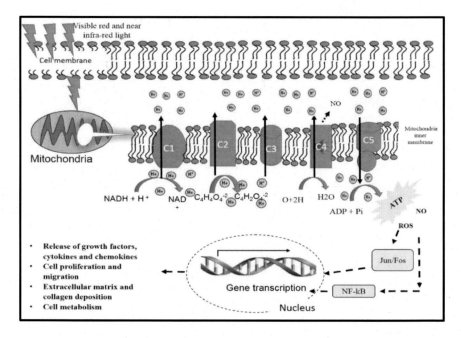

Figure 1. Mitochondrial unit IV (C4) of the respiratory chain is a chromophore and absorbs light in the visible red and near infra-red (NIR) light spectrum. This leads to increased mitochondrial membrane potential and electron translocation, giving rise to increased adenosine triphosphate (ATP), nitric oxide (NO) and reactive oxygen species (ROS) production. This in turn initiates transcription factors such as nuclear factor-kappa B (NF-κB), Jun and Fos, which translocates to the nucleus bringing about increased transcription of growth factors, cytokines and chemokines, resulting in increased cell proliferation, migration, extracellular matrix and collagen deposition and ultimately, increased wound healing.

The most critical aspect in any treatment method is the size or frequency or a level of exposure of a drug or radiation. The biostimulatory effects of PBM are most appreciated if used at the right parameters (energy density, power output, wavelength, pulse frequency and pulse duration) and exposure time. For instance, the correct amount of energy density depends on the medical disorder being treated, particularly the depth of tissue the light has to penetrate to reach its target. The optimal light penetration in the tissue and the wavelength absorbed by chromophores are the key limitations for consideration in PBMT, and the effective tissue penetration of light is maximised at wavelengths between 650 nm to

1200 nm (Silva et al. 2015; Hamblin, 2016). The inappropriate selection of these parameters may be the reason for negatory reports on the therapeutic effects of PBM (Rashidi et al. 2015). These conflicting reports and non-existence of consistency in therapeutic parameter optimisation makes PBMT to be underutilised in medicine (Ramos et al. 2018).

Photobiomodulation and Wound Healing

Many techniques are applied to stimulate wound healing, however, a large number of wounds remain unresponsive and difficult to heal using almost all the treatment options. The mystery of wound healing affects several biological processes at the tissue, cellular and molecular levels, and most research on wound healing focuses on cellular and subcellular biostimulation (Kajagar et al. 2012). Studies have shown that high blood glucose and acidosis interrupts the healing process of injured tissue. This process is able to be impeded by PBMT with no known side effects (Rashidi et al. 2015). The use and efficacy of PBMT for relegating inflammation, pain, and preventing tissue damage and stimulating wound healing is well documented (Rhee et al. 2017). The healing characteristics of PBMT are due to photobiostimulation, and results in the increased release of growth factors, increased cell migration, proliferation and differentiation, ECM and granulation tissue deposition, collagen synthesis, neoangiogenesis, and reepithelialisation. Low doses of PBMT are restorative while high doses have been found to be repressive (Kajagar et al. 2012). Disparities in treatment dosage and limits in experimental design have largely contributed to reports of no biostumulatory influence (Hopkins et al. 2004). Cellular, animal and randomised clinical studies demonstrate that wound healing is stimulated at different wavelengths and power densities with no conclusively defined optimal parameters. Although scientists believe that concurrent multiple wavelengths are effectual as compared to single wavelengths, the ideal wavelengths, single or multiple, needs to be clearly described for effective healing of both acute and chronic wounds (Kuffler, 2015).

In Vitro Studies

PBMT can stimulate dermal cell proliferation, migration and differentiation, collagen synthesis, angiogenesis and deposition of granulation tissue, and decrease the production of inflammatory cells (Ramos et al. 2019). Tricarico and colleagues (2018) assessed the influence of PBM in a human keratinocyte cell line (HaCaT cells) in promoting wound closure. Cells were irradiated with a diode laser at a wavelength of 970 nm, power density of 300 mW/cm^2 and a fluence of 60, 50, 40, 30, 20 and 10 J/cm^2. They noticed a significant time reduction for wound closure, with a significant increase in cell migration and ATP production at 2 hours. After 24 hours they noticed an upsurge in cellular metabolism with decreased levels of intracellular ATP. Solmaz and colleagues (2017) established that PBM at a wavelength of 635 nm with a fluence of 1 and 3 J/cm^2 and power output of 50 mW stimulates wound tensile strength, while a wavelength of 809 nm at the same fluencies and power output did not show any restorative outcome. Furthermore, they observed that at lower energy densities, PBM at a wavelength of 635 nm significantly increased cell proliferation and mechanistic strength of wounds *in vitro* and *in vivo*, respectively, with no positive effects at a wavelength of 809 nm with the same laser parameters. Rhee et al. (2017) used LED light at five different wavelengths namely 470 nm (blue light), 530 nm (green light), 660 nm (red light), 740 nm (red light), and 850 nm (NIR) on human corneal epithelial cells (HCE-T). They observed a significant decrease in cell survival at 470 nm, while at wavelengths greater than 660 nm PBM significantly influenced cell migration, with a wavelength of 740 nm being the most efficacious. The effect of different wavelengths on wound healing *in vitro* was also shown by de Abreu et al. (2019) and Houreld and Abrahamse (2008). de Abreu and colleagues conducted a review of the literature, and concluded that red and NIR light was more stimulatory on keratinocyte cells than blue light. Houreld and Abrahamse concluded that *in vitro* diabetic wounded fibroblast cells responded better to red and NIR light (632.8 nm and 830 nm, respectively) and at lower fluencies.

Amaroli et al. (2019) suggested that NIR light leads to a shift from anaerobic to aerobic metabolism in an *in vitro* scratch wound model using endothelial cells. NIR irradiation at 808 nm (output density of 1 W/cm^2, fluence of 60 J/cm^2) stimulated mitochondrial oxygen consumption, ROS production and ATP synthesis, as well as cellular migration and proliferation. The increase in ROS did not lead to an increase in oxidative stress nor oxidative stress-activated processes. PBM has been found to have anti-inflammatory effects on cells. Lim and colleagues (2015) irradiated immortalised human gingival fibroblasts (IGFs) in the presence of porphyromonas gingivalis lipopolysaccharides (LPS), one of the major pathogenic factors of chronic periodontitis. Cells were directly irradiated at a wavelength of 635 nm or indirectly irradiated whereby media from irradiated cells were added to non-irradiated cells. Inflammatory markers cyclooxygenase-2 (COX2) and prostaglandin E_2 (PGE_2) decreased post-irradiation in both direct and indirect irradiated cultures (Lim et al. 2015). In a similar study by the same group, irradiation of hypoxic human endothelial cells at 635 nm with a power density of 5 mW/cm^2 led to the reduced production and increased scavenging of intracellular ROS. There was increased vascular endothelial growth factor (VEGF) and VEGF receptor 1 (VEGFR-1) expression, which in-turn lead to the increased phosphorylation (activation) of ERK1/2 and mediation of MAPK signalling, resulting in accelerated angiogenesis and enhanced cell viability and tube formation (Lim et al. 2011).

Irradiation of diabetic wounded cells *in vitro* at a wavelength of 660 nm with a fluence of 5 J/cm^2 significantly speeds up wound healing. Irradiation has led to increased collagen production (Ayuk et al. 2012), increased gene expression of cellular adhesion molecules (Ayuk et al. 2016; Ayuk et al. 2014) and other ECM proteins (including collagen), as well as genes involved in the mitochondrial electron transport chain (Masha et al. 2013), increased cellular migration and proliferation via the JAK/STAT pathway (Jere et al. 2018), and a decrease in proteinases (Ayuk et al. 2014; Ayuk et al. 2018). Basso et al. (2013) also found an increase in collagen and VEGF when they irradiated keratinocytes at 780 ± 3 nm with 1.5 J/cm^2.

Animal Model Studies

Keshri et al. (2016) evaluated the photobiostimulatory outcomes on dermal wound healing using a diode laser at a wavelength of 810 nm, power density of 40 mW/cm^2 and fluence of 22.6 J/cm^2 with continuous and pulsed (10 and 100 Hz) wave light in immune suppressed rats. They noticed that PBM at a wavelength of 810 nm pulsed at 10 Hz significantly enhanced wound healing with decreased pro-inflammatory cytokines, and increased wound contraction, cell proliferation, neovascularisation, ECM deposition and reepithelialisation, and further upregulated the expression of proteins. Aimbire et al. (2006) found that PBMT at 650 nm and a power density of 31.3 mW/cm^2 reduced inflammation as determined by a reduction in tumour necrosis factor alpha (TNF-α) levels. Pigatto et al. (2019) irradiated mice at 660 nm (energy density of 84.64 mW/cm^2; fluencies of 2.531 J/cm^2, 5.07 J/cm^2, 7.61 J/cm^2, and 10.15 J/cm^2). Irradiation at a fluence of 5.07 J/cm^2 (60 seconds) led to a reduction of nociceptive neurogenic (1st phase) and inflammatory pain (2nd phase). There was also a decrease in the migration of inflammatory cells. Gupta et al. (2014) studied the healing effects of PBMT in the red and NIR wavelength spectrum (635, 730, 810 and 980 nm) delivered at a fluence of 4 J/cm^2 (10 mW/cm^2) in a mouse model of partial-thickness dermal abrasion. Wavelengths of 635 and 810 nm stimulated wound healing, while 730 and 980 nm produced no effects. The best results were observed at a wavelength of 810 nm, with a significant decrease in wound size, increased collagen accumulation and complete reepithelialisation. These results suggest that wound repair using PBMT is wavelength dependent. Naterstad et al. (2018) were able to show that PBMT at 810 nm (power output of 100 mW, energy of 3 J) was significantly better over commonly used anti-inflammatory agents diclofenac and dexamethasone, used in acute collagenase-induced tendinitis in Wistar rats. Assis and colleagues (2012) showed that PBMT at 808 nm reduced inflammation and oxidative stress in injured muscle in rats.

Studies using PBMT in diabetic animal models have also shown positive effects on healing. Akyol and Güngörmüş (2010) irradiated wounded diabetic Wistar rats at a wavelength of 808 nm with a power density of 0.1 W/cm^2. Histology results showed that PBMT increased reepithelialisation and fibroblast proliferation. Wound closure was significantly enhanced and there was a quicker resolution of the inflammatory phase. Al-Watban et al. (2009) concluded that PBMT using the appropriate parameters accelerates burn wounds in diabetic rats. Diabetic rats were subjected to a burn wound and irradiated three times a week with wavelengths of either 532, 633, 670, 810, and 980 nm and at fluencies of 5, 10, 20, and 30 J/cm^2. Better healing was seen with lasers in the visible spectrum (532, 633, and 670 nm). The reason for this was not investigated.

Clinical Studies

PBMT has proven to be effective in facilitating the contraction of wounds in diabetic patients (Kajagar et al. 2012). Compromised healing processes in diabetic wounds is related to diminished cellular proliferation, migration, synthesis of NO, growth factors, and collagen, and an increase in proteinases. The prolonged inflammatory phase is accompanied by an increase in oxidative stress with intensified cell death. Cells in diabetic ulcers have been shown to respond favourably when exposed to PBM, and cellular studies have shown an increase in cellular migration, proliferation, viability, growth factors, and gene regulation (Houreld, 2014). In a clinical trial conducted by de Alencar Fonseca Santos et al. (2018) they aimed at investigating the efficacy of PBMT at a wavelength of 660 nm, power output of 30 mW and fluence of 6 J/cm^2 on the healing process of chronic diabetic wounds. They observed a significant improvement in tissue repair in the treated group when compared with an untreated control group. In a randomised trial, Priyadarshini et al. (2018) used red light at a wavelength of 660 nm and fluence of 4-8 J/cm^2 for 20 minutes. After completing daily treatment for 15 days, treated diabetic foot ulcers showed complete wound healing in approximately 67% of grade 1 ulcers and 4% of grade 2 ulcers, and 97% of grade 2 ulcers improved to grade 1, with a significant decrease in mean area of the ulcer as compared to their controls.

Caetano et al. (2009) conducted a randomised placebo-controlled double-blind study on 20 patients with 32 chronic ulcers that were larger than 1.0 cm^2, and that had persisted for more than six weeks. Patients were randomly assigned to one of three groups. Ulcers in group 1 were cleaned and dressed with 1% silver sulfadiazine (SDZ) cream and received placebo PBMT. Ulcers in group 2 were similarly cleaned and dressed, and received PBMT with a LED probe which consisted of 32 15 mW diodes at a wavelength of 890 nm, and 4 5 mW diodes at a wavelength of 600 nm. A total output power of 500 mW and a fluence of 3 J/cm^2 was used. Ulcers in group 3 were cleaned and dressed with SDZ cream (controls). Ulcers were treated twice a week for 90 days. Ulcers in group 2 healed significantly faster than ulcers in group 3 at 30, 60 and 90 days of evaluation. Even ulcers in group 1 healed quicker than ulcers in group 3, but only on day 90. Ulcers in group 1 received placebo PBMT, with the 890 nm diodes disabled, as well as three of the four 660 nm diodes. The power in the remaining 660 nm diode was significantly reduced and emitted light at less than 5 mW. The results showed that even long term exposure to very low powered light (less than 5 mW) offered some therapeutic benefit. Significant differences between groups 2 and 3 were still observed when only medium and large ulcers were compared (small ulcers healed completely before the 90-day treatment period was up). It was concluded that PBMT promotes healing of chronic, nonresponsive venous ulcers.

Cabras et al. (2016) reported on a case study whereby PBMT was used to treat persistent oral ulcerations as a result of long-term usage of hydroxyurea for the treatment of polycythemia vera. The patient was treated twice a week with a diode laser (GaAlAs) with a wavelength of 810 nm (100 mW and 6 J/cm^2) at a distance of 2 mm from the mucosa. Only after two weeks (four treatments) a pronounced improvement was observed. There was reepithelialisation of the mucosa together with the disappearance of pain. After another four weeks of PBMT topical corticosteroid treatment was stopped, and after another three weeks of PBMT symptoms and mucosal lesions were completely healed, together with functional recovery of the tongue. PBMT was shown to stimulate healing of otherwise non-responsive mucosal ulcers and alleviate pain associated with the ulcers, without any adverse effects.

Beckmann et al. (2014) conducted a systematic literature review on the use of PBM on diabetic ulcers. Most of the clinical studies showed a possible benefit, however many of these studies were limiting and it's been suggested that due to the promising nature of these studies, better and well-designed clinical studies should be conducted to authenticate the value and usefulness of PBMT. Overwhelming evidence on the therapeutic effects of PBMT on wound healing is still emerging, and based upon this, additional research may allow for persuasive endorsement of PBMT for wound healing.

CONCLUSION

Chronic wounds are undoubtedly a global epidemic, and wound care is becoming an important WHO initiative. Present opportunities for successful treatment of chronic wounds is limited and frequently associated with failure and relapse, and since chronic healing is associated with a prolonged inflammatory response, there is a pressing need to ascertain a reliable and safe treatment that incorporates all parameters involving inflammation and repair. Light in the visible red and near infrared range efficiently decreases inflammation and stimulates wound healing. PBMT at suitable dose limitations can enhance healing in chronic wounds. However, there are still several questions remaining to be answered. The precise cellular and molecular mechanisms of PBMT, the influential parameters and its effectiveness on distinctive chronic wounds are some of the key questions that may demand more research.

REFERENCES

Aimbire, F., Albertini, R., Pacheco, M. T. T., Castro-Faria-Neto, H. C., Leonardo, P. S. L. M., Iversen, V. V., Lopes-Martins, R. A. B. and

Bjordal, J. M. (2006). Low-Level Laser Therapy Induces Dose-Dependent Reduction of TNF Levels in Acute Inflammation. *Photomedicine and Laser Surgery*, 24: 33–37.

Akyol, U. and Gűngörműş, M. (2010). The Effect of Low-Level Laser Therapy on Healing of Skin Incisions Made Using a Diode Laser in Diabetic Rats. *Photomedicine and Laser Surgery*, 28: 51–55.

Al-Watban, F. A. H., Zhang, X. Y., Andres, B. L. and Al-Anize, A. (2009). Visible Lasers Were Better Than Invisible Lasers in Accelerating Burn Healing on Diabetic Rats. *Photomedicine and Laser Surgery*, 27: 269–272.

Amaroli, A., Ravera, S., Baldini, F., Benedicenti, S., Panfoli, I. and Vergani, L. (2019). Photobiomodulation with 808-nm diode laser light promotes wound healing of human endothelial cells through increased reactive oxygen species production stimulating mitochondrial oxidative phosphorylation. *Lasers in Medical Science*, 34: 495-504.

Assis, L., Moretti, A., Abrahão, T. B., Cury, V., Souza, H. P., Hamblin, M. R. and Parizotto, N. A. (2012). Low-level laser therapy (808 nm) reduces inflammatory response and oxidative stress in rat tibialis anterior muscle after cryolesion. *Lasers in Surgery and Medicine*, 44: 726-735.

Ayuk, S., Abrahamse, H. and Houreld, N. N. (2016). The role of photobiomodulation on gene expression of cell adhesion molecules in diabetic wounded fibroblasts *in vitro*. *Journal of Photochemistry and Photobiology, B: Biology*, 161: 368–374.

Ayuk, S., Abrahamse, H. and Houreld, N. N. (2018). Photobiomodulation alters matrix protein activity in stressed fibroblast cells *in vitro*. *Journal of Biophotonics*, 2018, 11. doi:10.1002/jbio.201700127.

Ayuk, S., Houreld, N. N. and Abrahamse, H. (2012). Collagen production in diabetic wounded fibroblasts in response to Low-Intensity Laser Irradiation at 660nm. *Diabetes Technology and Therapeutics*, 14: 1110-1117.

Ayuk, S., Houreld, N. N. and Abrahamse, H. (2014). Laser irradiation alters the expression profile of genes involved in the extracellular matrix i*n vitro. International Journal of Photoenergy.* Accessed July 4, 2019. doi:10.1155/2014/604518.

Basso, F. G., Oliveira, C. F., Kurachi, C., Hebling, J. and de Souza Costa, C. A. (2013). Biostimulatory effect of low-level laser therapy on keratinocytes *in vitro. Lasers in Medical Science*, 28: 367–374.

Beckmann, K. H., Meyer-Hamme, G. and Schröder, S. (2014). Low Level Laser Therapy for the Treatment of Diabetic Foot Ulcers: A Critical Survey. *Evidence-Based Complementary and Alternative Medicine*, 626127. Accessed July 4, 2019. doi:10.1155/2014/626127.

Bitar, M. S. (2012). The GSK-3beta/Fyn/Nrf2 pathway in fibroblasts and wounds of type 2 diabetes: on the road to an evidence-based therapy of non-healing wounds. *Adipocyte*, 1: 161–163.

Cabras, M., Cafaro, A., Gambino, A., Broccoletti, R., Romagnoli, E., Marina, D. and Arduino, P. G. (2016). Laser Photobiomodulation for a Complex Patient with Severe Hydroxyurea-Induced Oral Ulcerations. *Case Reports in Dentistry*, 9810480. Accessed July 4, 2019. doi:10.1155/2016/9810480.

Caetano, K. S., Frade, M. A. C., Minatel, D. G., Santana, L. Á. and Enwemeka, C. S. (2009). Phototherapy Improves Healing of Chronic Venous Ulcers. *Photomedicine and Laser Surgery*, 27: 111–118.

de Abreu, P. T. R., de Arruda, J. A. A., Mesquita, R. A., Abreu, L. G., Diniz, I. M. A. and Silva, T. A. (2019). Photobiomodulation effects on keratinocytes cultured *in vitro*: a critical review. *Lasers in Medical Science*, Accessed July 4, 2019. doi: 10.1007/s10103-019-02813-5.

de Alencar Fonseca Santos, J., Campelo, M. B. D., de Oliveira, R. A., Nicolau, R. A., Rezende, V. E. A. and Arisawa, E. Â. L. (2018). Effects of Low-Power Light Therapy on the Tissue Repair Process of Chronic Wounds in Diabetic Feet. *Photomedicine and Laser Surgery*, 36: 298–304.

De Freitas, L. F. and Hamblin, M. R. (2016). Proposed Mechanisms of Photobiomodulation or Low-Level Light Therapy. *IEEE Journal of Selected Topics in Quantum Electronics*, 22: Accessed June 11, 2019. doi: 10.1109/JSTQE.2016.2561201.

Demidova-Rice, T. N., Hamblin, M. R. and Herman, I. M. (2012). Acute and impaired wound healing: pathophysiology and current methods for drug delivery, part 1: normal and chronic wounds: biology, causes, and approaches to care. *Advances in Skin and Wound Care*, 25: 304–314.

Frykberg, R. G. and Banks, J. (2015). Challenges in the Treatment of Chronic Wounds. *Advances in Wound Care*, 4: 560-582.

Gonzalez, A. C., Costa, T. F., de Araújo Andrade, Z. and Medrado, A. R. A. P. (2016). Wound healing - A literature review. *Anais Brasileiros de Dermatologia*, 91: 614-620.

Gupta, A., Dai, T. and Hamblin, M. R. (2014). Effect of red and near infrared wavelengths on low-level laser (light) therapy induced healing of partial-thickness dermal abrasion in mice. *Lasers Medical Science*, 29: 257-265.

Hamblin, M. R. (2010). Introduction to Experimental and Clinical Studies Using Low-Level Laser (Light) Therapy (LLLT). *Lasers in Surgery and Medicine*, 42: 447–449.

Hamblin, M. R. (2016). Photobiomodulation or low-level laser therapy. *Journal of Biophotonics*, 9: 1122-1124.

Hamblin, M. R., Ferraresi, C., Huang, Y-Y., de Freitas, L. F. and Carroll, J. D. (2018). *Low-Level Light Therapy: Photobiomodulation*. SPIE Press ISBN: 9781510614154.

Han, G. and Ceilley, R. (2017). Chronic Wound Healing: A Review of Current Management and Treatments. *Advances in Therapy*, 34: 599–610.

Hopkins, J. T., McLoda, T. A., Seegmiller, J. G. and Baxter, G. D. (2004). Low-Level Laser Therapy Facilitates Superficial Wound Healing in Humans: A Triple-Blind, Sham-Controlled Study. *Journal of Athletic Training*, 39: 223–229.

Houreld, N. N. (2014). Shedding Light on a New Treatment for Diabetic Wound Healing: A Review on Phototherapy. *The Scientific World Journal*, 398412. Accessed July 4, 2019. doi:10.1155/2014/398412.

Houreld, N. N. and Abrahamse, H. (2008). Laser light influences cellular viability and proliferation in diabetic-wounded fibroblast cells in a dose- and wavelength-dependent manner. *Lasers in Medical Science*, 23: 11–18.

Houreld, N. N., Masha, R. T. and Abrahamse, H. (2012). Low-Intensity Laser Irradiation at 660 nm Stimulates Cytochrome c Oxidase in Stressed Fibroblast Cells. *Lasers in Surgery and Medicine*, 44: 429–434.

Järbrink, K., Ni, G., Sönnergren, H., Schmidtchen, A., Pang, C., Bajpai, R. and Car, J. (2017). The humanistic and economic burden of chronic wounds: a protocol for a systematic review. *Systematic Reviews*, 6: Accessed June 10, 2019. doi:10.1186/s13643-016-0400-8.

Jere, S. W., Houreld, N. N. and Abrahamse, H. (2018). Photobio-modulation at 660 nm stimulates proliferation and migration of diabetic wounded cells via the expression of epidermal growth factor and the JAK/STAT pathway. *Journal of Photochemistry and Photobiology, B: Biology*, 179: 74–83.

Jere, S. W., Houreld, N. N. and Abrahamse, H. (2019). Role of the PI3K/AKT (mTOR and GSK3β) signalling pathway and photobiomodulation in diabetic wound healing. *Cytokine and Growth Factor Reviews*. Accessed March 13, 2019. doi:10.1016/j.cytogfr.2019.03.001.

Kajagar, B. M., Godhi, A. S., Pandit, A. and Khatri, S. (2012). Efficacy of low level laser therapy on wound healing in patients with chronic diabetic foot ulcers-a randomised control trial. *The Indian Journal of Surgery*, 74: 359–363.

Keshri, G. K., Gupta, A., Yadav, A., Sharma, S. K. and Singh, S. B. (2016). Photobiomodulation with Pulsed and Continuous Wave Near-Infrared Laser (810 nm, Al-Ga-As) Augments Dermal Wound Healing in Immunosuppressed Rats. *PLoS ONE*, 11: e0166705. Accessed July 4, 2019. doi:10.1371/journal.pone.0166705.

Kohale, B. R., Agrawal, A. A. and Raut, C. P. (2018). Effect of low-level laser therapy on wound healing and patients' response after scalpel gingivectomy: A randomized clinical split-mouth study. *Journal of Indian Society of Periodontology*, 22: 419–426.

Kuffler, D. P. (2015). Photobiomodulation in promoting wound healing: a review. *Regenerative Medicine*, 11: 107-122.

Li, J., Chen, J. and Kirsner, R. (2007). Pathophysiology of acute wound healing. *Clinics in Dermatology*, 25: 9-18.

Lim, W. B., Kim, J. S., Ko, Y. J., Kwon, H., Kim, S. W., Min, H. K., Kim, O., Choi, H. R. and Kim, O. J. (2011). Effects of 635nm Light-Emitting Diode Irradiation on Angiogenesis in CoCl2-Exposed HUVECs. *Lasers in Surgery and Medicine*, 43: 344–352.

Lim, W., Choi, H., Kim, J., Kim, S., Jeon, S., Zheng, H., Kim, D., Ko, Y., Kim, D., Sohn, H. and Kim, O. (2015). Anti-inflammatory effect of 635 nm irradiations on *in vitro* direct/indirect irradiation model. *Journal of Oral Pathology and Medicine*, 44: 94-102.

Masha, R. T., Houreld, N. N. and Abrahamse, H. (2013). Low-Intensity Laser irradiation at 660nm stimulates transcription of genes involved in the electron transport chain. *Photomedicine and Laser Surgery*, 31: 47–53.

Naterstad, I. F., Rossi, R. P., Marcos, R. L., Parizzoto, N. A., Frigo, L., Joensen, J., Lopes Martins, P. S. L., Bjordal, J. M. and Lopes-Martins, R. A. B. (2018). Comparison of Photobiomodulation and Anti-Inflammatory Drugs on Tissue Repair on Collagenase-Induced Achilles Tendon Inflammation in Rats. *Photomedicine and Laser Surgery*, 36: 137-145.

Pigatto, G. R., Silva, C. S. and Parizzoto, N. A. (2019). Photobiomodulation therapy reduces acute pain and inflammation in mice. *Journal of Photochemistry and Photobiology, B: Biology*, 196: 111513. Accessed July 4, 2019. doi:10.1016/j.jphotobiol.2019.111513.

Priyadarshini, L. M. J., Babu, K. E. P. and Thariq, I. A. (2018). Effect of low level laser therapy on diabetic foot ulcers: a randomized control trial. *International Surgery Journal*, 5: 1008-1015.

Qing, C. (2017). The molecular biology in wound healing & non-healing wound. *Chinese Journal of Traumatology*, 20: 189–193.

Ramos, F. S., Maifrino, L. B. M., Alves, S., da Costa Aguiar Alves, B. Perez, M. M., Feder, D., Azzalis, L. A., Junqueira, V. B. C. and Fonseca, F. L. A. (2018). The effects of transcutaneous low-level laser therapy on the skin healing process: an experimental model. *Lasers in Medical Science*, 33: 967–976.

Ramos, R. M., Burland, M., Silva, J. B., Burman, L. M., Gelain, M. S., Debom, L. M., Bec, J. M. Alirezai, M., Uebel, C. O. and Valmier, J. (2019). Photobiomodulation improved the first stages of Wound healing process after abdominoplasty: An experimental, double-blinded, non-randomized clinical trial. *Aesthetic Plastic Surgery*, 43: 147–154.

Rashidi, S., Yadollahpour, A. and Mirzaiyan, M. (2015). Low Level Laser Therapy for the Treatment of Chronic Wound: Clinical Considerations. *Biomedical and Pharmacology Journal*, 8: 1121-1127.

Rhee, Y. H., Cho, K. J., Ahn, J. C. and Chung, P. S. (2017). Effect of Photobiomodulation on Wound Healing of the Corneal Epithelium through Rho-GTPase. *Medical Lasers; Engineering, Basic Research, and Clinical Application*, 6: 67-76.

Samaniego-Ruiz, M. J., Llatas, F. P. and Jiménez, O. S. (2018). Assessment of chronic wounds in adults: an integrative review. *Revista da Escola de Enfermagem da USP*, 52: e03315. Accessed June 10, 2019. doi:10.1590/S1980-220X2016050903315.

Silva, A. A., Leal-Junior, E. C., D'Avila Kde, A., Serra, A. J., Albertini, R., França, C. M., Nishida, J. A. and de Carvalho Pde, T. (2015). Pre-exercise low-level laser therapy improves performance and levels of oxidative stress markers in mdx mice subjected to muscle fatigue by high-intensity exercise. *Lasers in Medical Science*, 30: 1719-1727.

Solmaz, H., Ulgen, Y. and Gulsoy, M. (2017). Photobiomodulation of wound healing via visible and infrared laser irradiation. *Lasers in Medical Science*, 32: 903-910.

Sorg, H., Tilkorn, D. J., Hager, S., Hauser, J. and Mirastschijsk, U. (2017). Skin Wound Healing: An Update on the Current Knowledge and Concepts. *European Surgical Research*, 58: 81–94.

Tricarico, P. M., Zupin, L., Ottaviani, G., Pacor, S., Jean-Louis, F., Boniotto, M. and Crovella, S. (2018). Photobiomodulation therapy promotes *in vitro* wound healing in nicastrin KO HaCaT cells. *Journal of Biophotonics*, 11: e201800174. Accessed June 11, 2019. doi: 10.1002/jbio.201800174.

Turner, N. J. and Badylak, S. F. (2015). The Use of Biologic Scaffolds in the Treatment of Chronic Nonhealing Wounds. *Advances in Wound Care*, 4: 490–500.

World Health Organisation. (2010). *Wound and lymphoedema management*. Accessed July 11, 2019. http://whqlibdoc.who.int/ publications/2010/ 9789241599139_eng.pdf.

Zungu, I. L., Hawkins Evans, D. and Abrahamse, H. (2009). Mitochondrial Responses of Normal and Injured Human Skin Fibroblasts Following Low Level Laser Irradiation—An *In Vitro* Study. *Photochemistry and Photobiology*, 85: 987–996.

Biographical Sketches

Nicolette Houreld

Affiliation: Laser Research Centre, Faculty of Health Sciences, University of Johannesburg

Education: D.Tech Biomedical Technology

Research and Professional Experience: Research area of interest lies in photobiomodulation and diabetic wound healing, and investigates the molecular and cellular effects of photobiomodulation and laser tissue interaction.

Professional Appointments: Associate Professor

Honors: DST-NRF SARChI Deputy Chair-holder: Laser Applications in Health
C1 NRF rated scientist

Deputy Vice Chair of the faculty Research Ethics Committee

Editorial board Photobiomodulation, Photomedicine and Laser Surgery

Executive committee member World Association for photobiomoduLation Therapy (WALT)

Publications from the Last 3 Years:

[1]   Houreld, N. N. (2017). Are MIQE Guidelines Being Adhered to in qPCR Investigations in Photobiomodulation Experiments? *Photomedicine and Laser Surgery*, 35(2): 69-70.

[2]   Kruger, H., Khumalo, V. and Houreld, N. (2017). The prevalence of osteoarthritic symptoms of the hands amongst female massage therapists. *Health SA Gesondheid*, 22: 184-193.

[3]   Manoto, S., Hodgkinson, N, Houreld, N. and Abrahamse, H. (2017). Modes of cell death induced by Photodynamic therapy using Zinc Phthalocynaine in lung cancer cells grown as a monolayer and three dimensional multicellular tumour spheroids. *Molecules*, 22: 791, doi:10.3390/molecules22050791.

[4]   Jere, S., Abrahamse, H. and Houreld, N. (2017). Delayed wound healing: Ligand stimulation of the JAK/STAT signaling pathway and photobiomodulation. *Cytokine & Growth Factor Reviews*, 38: 73-79 https://doi.org/10.1016/j.cytogfr.2017.10.001.

[5]   Houreld, N. (2017). Mitochondrial light absorption and its effect on ATP production. In: MR Hamblin, T. Agrawal and M de Sousa (eds) Handbook of Low Level Laser Therapy. Pan Stanford Publishing, pp. 101-118. ISBN: 978-9814669603.

[6]   Ayuk, S., Abrahamse, H. and Houreld, N. (2018). Photobiomodulation alters matrix metalloproteinase activity. *Journal of Biophotonics*, 11(3): e201700127 DOI: 10.1002/jbio.201700127.

[7]   Mfouo-Tynga, I., Houreld, N. and Abrahamse, H. (2018). Characterization of a Multiple Particle Delivery Complex and Determination of Cellular Photodamage in Skin Fibroblast and Breast

Cancer Cell Lines. *Journal of Biophotonics*, 11(2): e201700077. doi: 10.1002/jbio.201700077.

[8]   Kumar, S. S. D., Houreld, N. N., Kroukamp, E. M. and Abrahamse, H. (2018). Cellular Imaging and Bactericidal Mechanism of Green-Synthesized Silver Nanoparticles against Human Pathogenic Bacteria. *Journal of Photochemistry & Photobiology, B: Biology*, 178: 259-269.

[9]   Kumar, S. S. D., Mahesh, M., Antoniraj, G., Rathore, H. S., Houreld, N. N. and Kandasamy, R. (2018). Cellular Imaging and Folate Receptor Targeting Delivery of Gum Kondagogu Capped Gold Nanoparticles in Cancer Cells. *International Journal of Biological Macromolecules*, 109: 220-230 https://doi.org/10.1016/ j.ijbiomac. 2017.12.069.

[10] Kumar, S. S. D., Houreld, N. N. and Abrahamse, H. (2018). Therapeutic Potential and Recent Advances of Curcumin in the Treatment of Aging-Associated Diseases. *Molecules*, 23: 835, doi:10.3390/molecules23040835.

[11] Kumar, S. S. D., Rajendran, N. K., Houreld, N. N. and Abrahamse, H. (2018). Recent Advances on silver nanoparticle based biomaterials and their application in wound healing. *International Journal of Biological Macromolecules*, 115: 165-175. https://doi.org/ 10.1016/ j.ijbiomac.2018.04.003.

[12] Jere, S. W., Houreld, N. N. and Abrahamse, H. (2018). Effect of photobiomodulation on the activation of the autocrine loop of epidermal growth factor/receptor through the Janus Kinase/Signal Transducer and Activators of Transcription pathway in diabetic wounded cells. *Journal of Photochemistry and Photobiology B: Biology*, 179: 74-83. doi:_10.1016/j.jphotobiol.2017.12.026.

[13] Rajendran, N. K., Kumar, S. S. D., Houreld, N. N. and Abrahamse, H. (2018). A Review on Nanoparticles Based Treatment for Wound Healing. *Journal of Drug Delivery Science and Technology*, 44: 421-430. doi.org/10.1016/j.jddst.2018.01.009.

[14] Ayuk, S. M., Houreld, N. N. and Abrahamse, H. (2018). Effect of 660 nm visible red light on cell proliferation and viability in diabetic

models *in vitro* under stressed conditions. *Lasers in Medical Science*, 33(5): 1085-1093. doi: 10.1007/s10103-017-2432-2.

[15] Houreld, N. N., Ayuk, S. M. and Abrahamse, H. (2018). Cell Adhesion Molecules are Mediated by Photobiomodulation at 660 nm in Diabetic Wounded Fibroblast Cells. *Cells*, 7: 30. doi:10.3390/cells7040030.

[16] Mfouo Tynga, I., Houreld, N. and Abrahamse, H. (2018). Evaluation of cell damage induced by irradiated Zinc-Phthalocyanine-gold dendrimeric particles in a breast cancer cell line. *Biomedical Journal*, 41: 254-264. doi.org/10.1016/j.bj.2018.05.002.

[17] Mokoena, D., Dhilip Kumar, S. S., Houreld, N. N. and Abrahamse, H. (2018). Role of Photobiomodulation on the Activation of the Smad Pathway via TGF-β in Wound Healing. *Journal of Photochemistry and Photobiology B: Biology*, 189: 138-144. https://doi.org/10.1016/j.jphotobiol.2018.10.011.

[18] Jere, S. W., Abrahamse, H. and Houreld, N. N. (2018). Photo-biomodulation activates the JAK/STAT signaling pathway in diabetic wounded cells *in vitro*. In: Proceedings of the 62nd annual conference of the South African Institute of Physics (SAIP2017). SAIP, South Africa, pp 199-203. ISBN 978-0-620-82077-6.

[19] Houreld, N. N. and Ayuk, S. M. (2018). Influence of Photo-biomodulation (Low-Level Laser Therapy) on Diabetic Wound Healing. In: V. Rai, J. Abdo, and S. Agrawal (Eds) *Low-Level Laser Therapy: History, Mechanisms, and Medical Uses*. Nova Biomedical, New York, USA, pp. 29-46. ISBN: 978-1-53613-2274.

[20] Abrahamse, H., Kumar, S. S. D. and Houreld, N. N. (2018). The Potential Role of Photobiomodulation and Polysaccharide Based Biomaterials in Wound Healing Applications. In: Turksen K. (Ed) *Wound Healing: Stem Cells Repair and Restorations, Basic and Clinical Aspects*. Wiley-Blackwell, pp. 211-223. ISBN: 978-1-119-28248-8 DOI: 10.1002/9781119282518.ch16.

[21] Rajendran, N. K., Dhilip Kumar, S. S., Houreld, N. N. and Abrahamse, H. (2019). Understanding the perspectives of forkhead transcription factors in wound healing and oxidative stress. *Journal of Cell Communication and Signalling*, 13: 151–162. https://doi.org/10.1007/s12079-018-0484-0.

[22] Gavish, L. and Houreld, N. N. (2019). Therapeutic Efficacy of Home-Use Photobiomodulation Devices – A Systematic Literature Review. *Photobiomodulation, Photomedicine, and Laser Surgery*, 37(1): 4-16. doi: 10.1089/photob.2018.4512.

[23] Houreld, N. N. (2019). The use of lasers and light sources in skin rejuvenation. *Clinics in Dermatology*, 37: 358-364. https://doi.org/10.1016/j.clindermatol.2019.04.008.

[24] Shaikh-Kader, A., Houreld, N. N., Rajendran, N. K. and Abrahamse, H. (2019). The link between advanced glycation end products and apoptosis in delayed wound healing. *Cell Biochemistry & Function*, 37: 432-442. DOI: 10.1002/cbf.3424.

[25] Abrahamse, H. and Houreld, N. N. (2019). Genetic aberrations associated with photodynamic therapy in colorectal cancer cells. *International Journal of Molecular Sciences*, 20: 3254. doi: 10.3390/ijms20133254.

[26] Jere, S. W., Houreld, N. N. and Abrahamse, H. (2019). The PI3K/AKT signalling pathway and effects of photobiomodulation in diabetic wound healing. *Cytokines and Growth Factor Reviews*. https:// doi.org/10.1016/j.cytogfr.2019.03.001.

[27] Thomas, M. M. and Houreld, N. N. (2019). The "in's and outs" of laser hair removal: a mini review. *Journal of Cosmetic and Laser Therapy*. In Press https://doi.org/10.1080/14764172.2019.1605449.

[28] Kumar, S. S. D., Houreld, N. N. and Abrahamse, H. (2019). Biopolymer-Baser Composites for Medical Applications. In: Hashmi, S. and Choudhury, I., (Eds) Reference Module in Materials Science and Materials Engineering, Elsevier, Oxford ISBN 978-0-12-813195-4. doi:10.1016/B978-0-12-803581-8.10557-0.

Sandy Winfield Jere

Affiliation: Laser Research Centre, Faculty of Health Sciences, University of Johannesburg

Education: M.Tech Biomedical Technology

Research and Professional Experience: 2010-2015, Civil servant (Medical Research Laboratory Technologist), Ministry of Health, Malawi. 2016-2020, Laser Research Centre, University of Johannesburg, South Africa, postgraduate student.

Professional Appointments: Current Doctoral student

Honors: Distinction M Tech

Publications from the Last 3 Years:

[1]   Jere, S. W., Houreld, N. N. and Abrahamse, H. (2019). Role of the PI3K/AKT (mTOR and GSK3β) signalling pathway and photobiomodulation in diabetic wound healing. *Cytokine and Growth Factor Reviews*, 19: 13-19.

[2]   Jere, S. W., Houreld, N. N. and Abrahamse, H. (2018). Photobiomodulation at 660 nm stimulates proliferation and migration of diabetic wounded cells via the expression of epidermal growth factor and the JAK/STAT pathway. *J. Photochem. Photobiol.*, 179: 74–83.

[3]   Jere, S. W., Abrahamse, H. & Houreld, N. N. (2018). Photobiomodulation activates the JAK/STAT signalling pathway in diabetic wounded cells *in vitro*. In: *SAIP 2017 Conference Proceeding.*, pp. 199-203. ISBN 978-0-620-82077-6.

[4]   Jere, S. W., Abrahamse, H. and Houreld, N. N. (2017). The JAK/STAT signaling pathway and photobiomodulation in chronic wound healing. *Cytokine and Growth Factor Reviews*, 38: 73–79.

In: A Closer Look at Wound Infections …   ISBN: 978-1-53616-816-7
Editor: Joseph E. Keel   © 2020 Nova Science Publishers, Inc.

Chapter 5

MANAGEMENT OF SURGICAL WOUNDS INFECTIONS IN SPINE SURGERY

M. Dobran[1], D. Nasi[1], S. Veccia[2] and A. Giacometti[2]
[1]Neurosurgery Clinic, Polytechnic University of Marche, Ancona, Italy
[2]Infectious Diseases Clinic, Polytechnic University of Marche,
Ancona, Italy

ABSTRACT

Postoperative surgical wound infection (SWI) in the lumbar spine is unfortunately a common and potentially devastating complication. It is associated with increasing morbidity and the need for further surgery.

The rate of spinal wound infection in literature ranges from 0.7 to 11.9% . The type of surgery is perhaps the most significant variable affecting the rate of infection. When instrumentation is used for lumbar fusions, the infection rate increases and Staphylococcus aureus is the most common organism causing SWI. Other reported causative organisms include Staphylococcus epidermidis, Enterococcus faecalis, Pseudomonas spp., Enterobacter cloacae and Proteus mirabilis. Gram-negative bacteria are more common in trauma patients. White blood cell count is an unreliable indicator of infection. Erythrocyte sedimentation rate (ESR) may remain elevated for up to six weeks after surgery and C-reactive protein (CRP) levels normalize within two weeks. In regard to the potential role of Procalcitonine (PCT), recent trials demonstrated that PCT may be useful to diagnose neurosurgical patients with SWI.

Magnetic resonance imaging (MRI) is the most useful study to diagnose SWI. Gadolinium enhancement improves the diagnostic accuracy of MRI and it should be used whenever an infection is suspected. Rim enhancing fluid collections, ascending epidural collections, the evidence of bone destruction and progressive marrow signal changes are suggestive of infection. The nonoperative treatment of postoperative spinal wound infections is rarely indicated and it is generally limited to significantly immunocompromised patients.

Treatment of SWI is centered on the surgical debridement of all necrotic tissue and the obtainment of intra-operative cultures to guide antibiotic therapy. We recommend the involvement of an infectious disease specialist to adjust and monitor the efficacy of the antibiotic treatment. In most cases, SWI can be adequately treated while leaving spinal instrumentation in place. For severe SWI, repeat debridements, delayer closure and the involvement of a plastic surgeon may be necessary. In some patients the use of the VAC therapy may be useful for the wound closure. Proven methods to prevent wound infection include prophylactic antibiotics, meticulous adherence to aseptic technique, frequent release of retractors to prevent myonecrosis and shorter operative time.

Keywords: surgical wound infections; spine surgery; antibiotic; surgical debridement

INTRODUCTION

Postoperative surgical wound infection (SWI) in the lumbar spine is unfortunately a common and potentially devastating complication [1]. It is associated with increased morbidity and the need for further surgery [2]. Additionally, the increasing prevalence of antibiotic-resistant organisms such as methicillin-resistant Staphylococcus aureus (MRSA) presents new challenges for both prevention and treatment of SWI, especially in patients with spinal instrumentation [3]. In this chapter, we review the epidemiology, the clinical presentation, the diagnosis and management of SWI.

EPIDEMIOLOGY

The rate of spinal wound infection in literature ranges from 0.7 to 11.9% [4]. The type of surgery is perhaps the most significant variable affecting the rate of infection. Simple lumbar discectomy carries a risk of infection of less than 1% thanks to shorter operative times, minor muscle trauma and generally healthier patients than those requiring more extensive spinal procedures [5]. When more extensive decompression is performed, with no fusion, the risk of infection increases from 1.5 to 2% [5]. With the addition of fusion to the procedure, operative time becomes longer, blood loss is greater and a separate operative site is usually required to harvest bone graft. The overall complication rate associated with a separate bone graft site is nearly 20%, some of them due to infection [6]. When instrumentation is used for lumbar fusions, the infection rate escalates from 2 to 6% [7].

Koutsoumbelis et al. [8] recently reviewed a consecutive series of 3,218 patients who underwent posterior lumbar instrumented arthrodesis. The surgery-related risk factors identified by their study included: (1) the presence of more than ten people in the operating room (OR), specifically cautioning against the presence of extraneous staff; (2) the long duration of surgery; (3) great intra-operative blood loss, the need for transfusion and (4) incidental durotomy.

Regarding patient-related risk factors for SWI, several studies reported the following factors: smoking, diabetes mellitus, alcohol abuse, obesity, malnutrition, advanced age, pre-operative hospitalization longer than one week and corticosteroid use. Smoking and diabetes have been shown to predispose patients to infection by inducing tissue ischemia and microvascular damage [9-11]. The thick layer of adipose tissue in obese patients provides a large potential space following surgical wound closure, which has poor vascular perfusion and may become necrotic.

Staphylococcus aureus is the most common organism causing SWI [12]. Recently, however, MRSA has become increasingly prevalent with 34% of SWIs according to the positive cultures in the series by Koutsoumbelis et al. [8]. Other reported causative organisms include

Staphylococcus epidermidis, Enterococcus faecalis, Pseudomonas spp., Enterobacter cloacae and Proteus mirabilis. Gram-negative bacteria are more common in trauma patients.

PREVENTION

The meticulous adherence to aseptic technique is the single most important component of SWI prevention [13]. The use of prophylactic antibiotic therapy has significantly decreased the rate of SWI after spinal surgery. Finally, frequent release of retractors to prevent myonecrosis, debridement of any necrotic appearing muscle and irrigation at the end of the procedure are recommended [14].

CLINICAL PRESENTATION

The overall diagnosis of SWI must be made using clinical judgment and taking into account any available information. SWI can be defined according to his anatomic relationship to the fascia (superficial or deep). In the early postoperative period, the most common signs of infection are increasing pain at the surgical site, open wound, metal protruding through skin, prominent metal ware, abscess and fluctuant wound. Objective findings on examination include peri-incisional erythema, tenderness to palpation, induration and drainage. Constitutional symptoms such as fever or chills are especially concerning revealing clues.

DIAGNOSIS

White blood cell count is an unreliable indicator of infection. The acute phase reactants are more useful to diagnose infection, but they must be interpreted. Erythrocyte sedimentation rate (ESR) may remain elevated for up to six weeks after surgery. C-reactive protein (CRP) levels normalize within two weeks. Consequently, CRP has been shown to be a more sensitive indicator of the presence of SWI [15].

In regard to the potential role of Procalcitonine (PCT), recent trials demonstrated that PCT may be useful in the diagnosis of neurosurgical patients with post-operative fever. Nevertheless other authors showed that CRP is more sensitive compared to PCT in patients with SWI [16].

Plain radiographs of the spine are rarely useful for the diagnosis of early infection. In the setting of discitis, there may be evidence of disc height loss and end plate erosion. In latent infections, lucencies may be present around the hardware. Magnetic resonance imaging (MRI) is the most useful study to diagnose SSI. Gadolinium enhancement improves the diagnostic accuracy of MRI and it should be used whenever an infection is suspected. Rim enhancing fluid collections, ascending epidural collections, evidence of bony destruction and progressive marrow signal changes are all suggestive of infection.

MANAGEMENT

Today titanium instrumentation in spine surgery grants an advantage: titanium alloy is less prone to colonization than stainless steel. Titanium is handy and widely used in spinal stabilization in traumatic and degeneratives pathologies of the column. In vitro studies suggest that the biofilm can block antibiotics, phagocytes and other humoral immune responders, making the infection relatively resistant to host defensive mechanisms and antibiotics. When a wound infection occurs in stabilized patients, the nonoperative treatment is rarely indicated and it is generally limited to significantly immunocompromised patients following an initial procedure involving irrigation and debridement to allow open-wound healing by means of secondary intention, dressing changes and wound packing.

Eradication of infection, however, nearly always requires careful debridement. Debate continues in literature about the need of serial debridements and their correct technique, if any, to close the skin and the fascial defect.

Debridement should consist of aggressive removal of all necrotic tissue and foreign materials such as sutures. Once the superficial layer has been debrided and irrigated copiously, the fascial layer must be inspected. This may be left unopened only if the surgeon is totally sure that the infection is only superficial. Once the deep layer is opened, debridement of necrotic muscle and significantly necrotic bone graft should be performed. In our experience and in literature, the leading philosophy is not to remove consolidating bone graft and instrumentation unless the infection is not healing in spite of debridements [1-5;16,17]. Instrumentation serves to stabilize the motion segment, theoretically decreasing inflammation and promoting bone healing. Some authors do not agree with leaving instrumentation in a contaminated wound. Non-essential spinal instrumentation such as loose pedicle screws should be removed. Anyway infection increases the risk of developing a pseudarthorosis and these patients must be closely monitored with serial imaging studies [18]. In cases of late infection with a solid fusion, instrumentation can be removed at the time of surgical debridement to facilitate the clearance of the infection.

Intra-operative tissue culture is essential to tailor antibiotic therapy before giving any. Close blood sugar control in diabetic patients and a nutrition consult in patients at risk for malnutrition are recommended [19-25].

It is a standard practice at our Institution to involve infectious disease specialists in the selection and serial monitoring of antibiotic therapy for SWI or other post-operative infections [26-28]. The antibiotic regimen is designed and monitored by an infectious disease specialist and based on the type of infectious organism and its drug sensitivity profile.

Intravenous antibiotic therapy is continued for at least six weeks postoperatively. In case of resistant organisms, such as MRSA, recent recommendations suggest extending intravenous antibiotic therapy for eight weeks [25]. At the end of the intravenous antibiotic therapy, we routinely maintain patients on oral suppressive antibiotics tailored to the infectious organism. The decision regarding the removal of the instrumentation versus life-time oral antibiotic suppression is based on the causative pathogen, the patient's health status and the presence of a fusion mass. Recently, vacuum-assisted closure of postoperative spinal wounds after infection has gained in popularity, although only isolated reports have appeared in literature. This technique consist of an occlusive dressing over a suction drainage system. The vacuum effect draws the edges of the wound together removing any purulent tissue. Success has been reported on a limited basis, but further trials need to be performed to determine any potential benefit compared with repeated debridement and tertiary closure or flap closures.

The necessary debridement of necrotic tissue following SWI may result in a significant soft tissue defect repaired with a muscle flap. This allows for high local antibiotic concentrations despite poor tissue vascularity. Multiple debridements are usually necessary and we recommend involvement of a plastic surgeon at early stage to grant an optimal wound management. Until today multiple techniques have been used for delayed wound closure. Negative pressure wound therapy (vacuum-assisted closure VAC) has been widely used for many years to treat complicated wounds and in case of failure of any surgical procedure. In many patients VAC therapy, also in presence of a wound infection, allowed the healing of the wound without removing the hardware. This is in line with the current trend to maintain the hardware in infected patients too.

In a recent study [28] we reviewed retrospectively 550 patients who underwent spinal fusion surgery from 2011 to 2015; 16 developed SSI after spinal instrumentation. The diagnosis of SWI was established according to positive wound swab or blood cultures and several clinical, laboratory and radiological findings. Additional pre-operative and intraoperative risk factors were analyzed. The incidence of SWI after spinal instrumentation surgery was 2.9%. Obesity was a statistically significant parameter ($p = 0,013$) that contributed to SWI along with alcoholism and/or drug abuse ($p = 0.034$).

The second study [27] on our patients documented that ESR and CRP values were statistically significant parameters to diagnose SWI after spinal implant. The leukocyte count, the number of lymphocytes and fever integrates the data of ESR and CRP with no statistical significance. MRI with contrast is the exam of choice, but FDG PET/CT may be useful in patients with a suspicion of SWI. Some pathogens have proved to be particularly hard to treat conservatively such as staphylococcus-MRSA. However some patients with SWI gain clinical healing with favorable outcome by means of target antibiotic therapy with no hardware removal.

In regard to the potential role of Procalcitonine (PCT), recent trials demonstrated that PCT may be useful to diagnose neurosurgical patients with post-operative fever. Nevertheless other authors showed that CRP is more sensitive than PCT in patients with SWI [15,16].

Plain radiographs of the spine are rarely useful to the diagnosis of early infection. In the setting of discitis there may be evidence of disc height loss and end plate erosion. In latent infections, lucencies may be present around the hardware. Magnetic resonance imaging (MRI) is the most useful study to diagnose SWI. Gadolinium enhancement improves the diagnostic accuracy of MRI and it should be used whenever an infection is suspected. Rim enhancing fluid collections, ascending epidural collections, the evidence of bony destruction and the progressive marrow signal changes are all suggestive of infection.

CONCLUSION

The treatment of SWI is centered on the surgical debridement of all necrotic tissue and the obtainment of intra-operative cultures to guide antibiotic therapy. We recommend the involvement of an infectious disease specialist to adjust and monitor the efficacy of antibiotic treatment. In most cases, SWI can be adequately treated while leaving spinal instrumentation in place. For severe SWI, repeated debridements, delayed closure and the involvement of a plastic surgeon are necessary. Proven methods to prevent wound infection include prophylactic antibiotics, meticulous adherence to aseptic technique, frequent release of retractors to prevent myonecrosis and shorter operative time. To prevent myonecrosis, debridement of any necrotic appearing muscle and the irrigation at the end of the procedure are recommended [14].

REFERENCES

[1] Weinstein MA, McCabe JP, Cammisa FP Jr (2000) Postoperative spinal wound infection: a review of 2,391 consecutive index procedures. *J. Spinal Disord.* 13:422–426.

[2] Bassewitz HL, Fischgrund JS, Herkowitz HN (2000) Postoperative spine infections. *Semin. Spine Surg.* 12:203–211.

[3] Weiner BK, Kilgore WB (2007) Bacterial shedding in common spine surgical procedures. *Spine* 32:918–920.

[4] National Nosocomial Infections Surveillance System (2004) National nosocomial infections surveillance (NNIS) system report, data summary from January 1992 through June 2004, issued October 2004. *Am. J. Infect. Control.* 32:470–485.

[5] Fang A, Hu SS, Endres N, Bradford DS (2005) Risk factors for infection after spinal surgery. *Spine* 30:1460–1465.

[6] Olsen MA, Mayfield J, Lauryssen C, Polish LB, Jones M, Vest J, Fraser VJ (2003) Risk factors for surgical site infection in spinal surgery. *J. Neurosurg.* 98(2 Suppl):149–155.

[7] Olsen MA, Nepple JJ, Riew KD, Lenke LG, Bridwell KH, Mayfield J, Fraser VJ (2008) Risk factors for surgical site infection following orthopaedic spinal operations. *J. Bone Joint Surg. Am.* 90:62–69.

[8] Koutsoumbelis S, Hughes AP, Girardi FP, Cammisa FP, Finerty EA, Nguyen JT, Gausden E, Sama AA (2011) Risk factors for postoperative infection following posterior lumbar instrumented arthrodesis. *J. Bone Joint Surg. Am.* 93:1627–1633.

[9] Carreon LY, Puno RM, Dimar JR 2nd, Glassman SD, Johnson JR (2003) Perioperative complications of posterior lumbar decom-

pression and arthrodesis in older adults. *J. Bone Joint Surg. Am.* 85:2089–2092.

[10] Cassinelli EH, Eubanks J, Vogt M, Furey C, Yoo J, Bohlman HH (2007) Risk factors for the development of perioperative complications in elderly patients undergoing lumbar decompression and arthrodesis for spinal stenosis: an analysis of 166 patients. *Spine* 32:230–235.

[11] Patel N, Bagan B, Vadera S, Maltenfort MG, Deutsch H, Vaccaro AR, Harrop J, Sharan A, Ratliff JK (2007) Obesity and spine surgery: relation to perioperative complications. *J. Neurosurg. Spine* 6:291–297.

[12] Levi AD, Dickman CA, Sonntag VK (1997) Management of postoperative infections after spinal instrumentation. *J. Neurosurg.* 86:975–980.

[13] Barker FG II (2002) Efficacy of prophylactic antibiotic therapy in spinal surgery: A meta-analysis. *Neurosurgery* 51:391–400.

[14] Transfeldt EE, Lonstein JE (1985) Wound infections in elective reconstructive spinal surgery. *Orthopaedic Transactions* 9:128–129.

[15] Silber JS, Anderson DG, Vaccaro AR, Anderson PA, McCormick P (2002) Management of post procedural discitis. *Spine J.* 2:279–287.

[16] Sierra-Hoffman M, Jinadatha C, Carpenter JL, Rahm M (2010) Postoperative instrumented spine infections: a retrospective review. *South Med. J.* 103:25–30.

[17] Pappou IP, Papadopoulos EC, Sama AA, Girardi FP, Cammisa FP (2006) Postoperative infections in interbody fusion for degenerative spinal disease. *Clin. Orthop. Relat. Res.* 444:120–128.

[18] Viola RW, King HA, Adler SA, Wilson CB (1997) Delayed infection after elective spinal instrumentation and fusion. A retrospective analysis of eight cases. *Spine* 22:2444–2450.

[19] Toulson C, Walcott-Sapp S, Hur J, Salvati E, Bostrom M, Brause B, Westrich GH (2009) Treatment of infected total hip arthroplasty with a 2-stage reimplantation protocol. *J. Arthroplasty* 24:1051–1060.

[20] Westrich GH, Walcott-Sapp S, Bornstein LJ, Bostrom MP, Windsor RE, Brause BD (2010) Modern treatment of infected total knee

arthroplasty with a 2-stage reimplantation protocol. *J. Arthroplasty* 25:1015–1021.

[21] Volin SJ, Hinrichs Sh, Garvin KL (2004) Two-stage reimplantation of total joint infections: a comparison of resistant and non-resistant organisms. *Clin. Orthop. Relat. Res.* 427:94–100.

[22] Weinstein MP, Stratton CW, Hawley HB, Ackley A, Reller LB (1987) Multicenter collaborative evaluation of a standardized se- rum bactericidal test as a predictor of therapeutic efficacy in acute and chronic osteomyelitis. *Am. J. Med.* 83:218–222.

[23] Liu C, Bayer A, Cosgrove SE et al. (2011) Clinical practice guidelines by the infectious diseases society of America for the treat- ment of methicillin-resistant *Staphylococcus aureus* infections in adults and children. *Clin. Infect. Dis.* 52:285–292.

[24] Mitra A, Mitra A, Harlin S (2004) Treatment of massive thoraco- lumbar wounds and vertebral osteomyelitis following scoliosis surgery. *Plast Reconstr. Surg.* 113:206–213.

[25] Dumanian GA, Ondra SL, Liu J, Schafer MF, Chao JD (2003) Muscle flap salvage of spine wounds with soft tissue defects or infection. *Spine* 28:1203–1211.

[26] Dobran M, Mancini F, Nasi D, Scerrati M (2017) A case of deep infection after instrumentation in dorsal spinal surgery: the management with antibiotics and negative wound pressure without removal of fixation. *BMJ Case Rep.* 28;2017.

[27] Dobran M, Marini A, Gladi M, Nasi D, Colasanti R, Benigni R, et al. (2017) Deep spinal infection in instrumented spinal surgery: diagnostic factors and therapy. *G Chir.* 38(3):124-129.

[28] Dobran M, Marini A, Nasi D, Gladi M, Liverotti V, Costanza MD et al. (2017) Risk factors of surgical site infections in instrumented spine surgery. *Surg. Neurol. Int.* 6;8:212.

INDEX

Index

C

N

O

P

R

S

Z

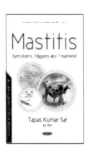

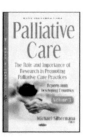
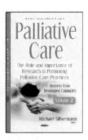